# Assessment of the Pulmonary Patient

# Assessment of the Pulmonary Patient

## Robin J. Dixon

**Assistant Professor**
**Department of Cardiopulmonary Care**
**Georgia State University**

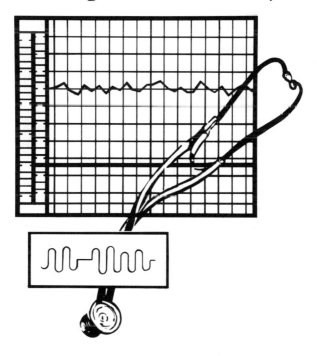

**Faculty Lecture Series
in Respiratory Care**

John W. Youtsey, Editor

**MULTI-MEDIA PUBLISHING, INC., BOOK DIVISION**
**1393 S. INCA STREET, DENVER, COLORADO 80223**

**Library of Congress Cataloging in Publication Data**

Dixon, Robin J., 1952-
    Assessment of the pulmonary patient.

    (Faculty lecture series in respiratory care)
    Bibliography: p.
    Includes index.
    1. Lungs—Diseases—Diagnosis. 2. Medical history
taking. 3. Physical diagnosis. I. Title. II. Series.
[DNLM: 1. Lung Diseases—diagnosis. WF 600 D621a]
RC733.D53 1985    616.2'407'54    84-43158
ISBN 0-940122-17-0

MMP/BC/BC  9 8 7 6 5 4 3 2 1

iv

# DEDICATION

This book is dedicated to the memory of Maxine.

## ABOUT THE AUTHOR

Robin J. Dixon is an assistant professor in the Department of Cardiopulmonary Care Sciences at Georgia State University in Atlanta, Georgia, where he has held a faculty position since 1979. He serves as the Director of Clinical Education for the Entry Level Practitioner Program at Georgia State. He has taught a variety of courses in both the entry level and advanced practitioner programs relating to basic respiratory therapy modalities and equipment, patient assessment, electrocardiography, airway management, neonatal and pediatric respiratory care, as well as intensive care clinical instruction. A graduate of Furman University, he received his Masters of Medical Sciences in Intensive Respiratory Care from Emory University School of Medicine, Atlanta, Georgia, in 1977.

Mr. Dixon has published in *Respiratory Care,* is co-author of a review text for respiratory therapy practitioners currently in press, and he serves as Editor of the Georgia Society for Respiratory Therapy Newsletter.

# TABLE OF CONTENTS

**Foreword   xii**

**Preface   xiii**

**Acknowledgments   xiv**

**Chapter 1: The Patient Interview   3**

Clinical Approach   3
Privacy   3
Initiating the interview   4
Attitude   4

Proper Questioning Techniques   6
Nonverbal communication   9

Listening   9

Potential Pitfalls   10

**Chapter 2: The Patient History   17**

Chief Complaint   17

History of Present Illness   17
Date of onset   18
Nature of complaint   18
Course of complaint   19
Location   19
Exacerbations   20
Treatment   20

Past Medical History   20
Childhood diseases   22
Previous hospitalizations   22
Accidents   23
Illnesses   23

Family History   23

Personal History   24

Life History   24

Socioeconomic Status   25

Occupational History   25

Education   25

Medications   25

Personal Habits   26

Smoking History   27

**Chapter 3: Cardiopulmonary Symptoms   31**

Cough   31
   Cough mechanism   31
   Pulmonary disease   32

Sputum   33
   Sputum production   34
   Sputum characteristics   35

Hemoptysis   35
   Trauma   36
   Inflammation   36
   Bronchiectasis   37
   Aspiration of foreign bodies   37
   Carcinoma   37
   Cardiovascular disease   37
   Source of hemoptysis   38

Dyspnea   38
   Cardiopulmonary disease   39
   Inspiratory and expiratory dyspnea   39
   Characterizing dyspnea   40
   Chronic obstructive pulmonary disease   42

Chest Pain   42
   Precordial pain   42
   Tracheobronchial pain   43
   Pleuritic pain   43
   Substernal pain   44
   Musculoskeletal pain   46

Characterizing Pain   46
   Palpitation   48

Wheezing   49
   Expiratory wheezes   50
   Evaluating wheezing   50

**Chapter 4: Approach to the Physical Examination   55**

Examination Procedure   55

Examination Room Environment   56

Measuring Vital Signs   57

Temperature   57

Pulse    62
  Rate    62
  Rhythm    63
  Character    63
  Abnormalities of the pulse    63

Blood Pressure    64
  Procedure    65
  Auscultory gap    65
  Normal findings    66
  Pulse pressure    66
  Mean arterial pressure    67
  Variations in blood pressure    67
  Sources of error in blood pressure measurement    68

**Chapter 5: Inspection    71**

Mental Status    72

Nutritional Status    73

Posture    74

Skin    74
  Color    75
  Cyanosis    75

Neck    76
  Size and shape    76
  Mobility    77
  Symmetry    77
  Scars    77
  Pulsations    78
  Laryngeal cartilages    78
  Accessory muscles of inspiration    78

Extremities    78
  Nails    79
  Digital clubbing    79
  Edema    81

Thorax    81
  Reference lines    81
  Bony landmarks    83
  Lobar anatomy    84
  Segmental anatomy of the lungs    88
  Inspection of the chest    89
  Thoracic deformities    90

Retractions and use of the accessory muscles
of inspiration   96

Rate, Type, and Pattern of Breathing   98

**Chapter 6: Palpation   103**

The Skin   103

The Neck   103
Laryngeal structures   103
Thyroid gland   104
Trachea   106

Thorax and Lungs   108
Thoracic expansion   108
Vocal (tactile) fremitus   111
Crepitations   112
Point of Maximal Impulse (PMI)   113

**Chapter 7: Percussion   117**

Techniques of Percussion   118

Characteristics of Percussion Notes   120

Pitch   120
Intensity   120
Duration   120
Quality   120

Percussion Notes and Their Location   121
Resonant percussion note   121
Hyperresonant percussion note   122
Tympanic percussion note   122
Dull percussion note   123
Flat percussion note   123

Diaphragmatic Excursion   124

**Chapter 8: Auscultation   129**

Auscultory Tones   129

The Stethoscope   130
Earpieces   130
Stethoscope tubing   131
Chest pieces   131

Technique of Auscultation   132

Errors in Auscultation   133

Normal Breath Sounds   134

Abnormal Breath Sounds   136
  Adventitious sounds   138

Voice Sounds   139

Heart Sounds   141
  First heart sound   141
  Second heart sound   141
  Ventricular ($S_3$) gallop   142
  Atrial ($S_4$) gallop   143
  Valve areas   143

**Chapter 9: Historical and Physical Findings in Specific Diseases   147**

Asthma   147

Emphysema   150

Chronic Bronchitis   153

Pneumonia   156

Pulmonary Fibrosis   158

Atelectasis   161

Pleural Effusion   164

Pneumothorax   167

**Bibliography**   173

**Index**   183

# FOREWORD

The field of respiratory therapy has progressed greatly in the past twenty years. In fact, it is no longer appropriate to refer to respiratory therapy as a field. The more correct word is profession.

Since the early 1960s, the respiratory therapist has evolved from obscure equipment specialist to mature health care practitioner. Recently, yet another milestone has occured in our professional development: Respiratory Care has replaced Respiratory Therapy as the official name of our discipline. With these changes comes a greater need for the respiratory care practitioner to have access to a wide selection of texts, monographs, and professional resources.

This text, *Assessment of the Pulmonary Patient,* is the first in a series entitled "The Faculty Lecture Series in Respiratory Care." This series typifies a new era in the development of text and reference books for respiratory care. The material presented in this book, as well as in those to follow, represents an effort to integrate the physiological basis of pulmonary medicine with its clinical application to patient care.

Often faculty find it very difficult to select appropriate textbooks for students. The ultimate goal in any text selection is to find that book which will be appropriate for the particular course(s) in the curriculum and yet will continue to be useful to the graduate as a clinical resource. Each book in this series will meet those goals.

In *Assessment of the Pulmonary Patient,* Robin Dixon has written a theoretically sound and clinically applicable book. He has successfully related interview techniques, chest assessment, and pulmonary pathophysiology to patient care. All health care practitioners who provide direct patient care will readily see the great value of Mr. Dixon's work.

—John W. Youtsey

Georgia State University
Atlanta, Georgia

xii

## PREFACE

*Assessment of the Pulmonary Patient,* a part of the Faculty Lecture Series in Respiratory Care, is a monograph on the components of a history and a chest physical examination of the patient with pulmonary disorders. It is intended to be used as an instructional tool by those health care professionals who see patients with pulmonary problems, namely respiratory care practitioners, nurse clinicians, medical students and pulmonary fellows. Although some physiology is highlighted, it is assumed the reader has a fundamental knowledge of pulmonary anatomy and diseases.

The first three chapters present the components of an accurate and complete pulmonary history. Chapter one describes how to conduct a patient interview with emphasis on questioning techniques designed to guide the patient through an informative interview. The second and third chapters discuss the questions which should be asked during the interview and symptoms which are common to patients with pulmonary problems.

Chapters four through eight deal with the physical examination of the patient, including: the measurement of vital signs, inspection, palpation, chest percussion and auscultation. Emphasis is placed on the origin of abnormal breath sounds and the proper terminology to use when describing breath sounds.

Chapter nine discusses common pulmonary diseases. The objective of this chapter is to make the reader aware of what to expect from the history and chest examination in specific diseases. The chapter concludes with a table summarizing the chest examination results of patients with various pulmonary disorders.

—Robin J. Dixon

## ACKNOWLEDGMENTS

This book would not have been possible without the support of my colleagues in the Department at Georgia State University, and especially the Chairman, Dr. John W. Youtsey who edited the manuscript and reminded me of deadlines. I also want to thank Albert K. Blackwelder, R.R.T. of Crawford W. Long Memorial Hospital, Atlanta, for his critical review of the manuscript.

I am grateful to Usha Saindane for the original artwork she supplied and to Alphonso Rosser in the Department of Public Information at Georgia State University who took the photographs. Additional artistic embellishments were provided by the Educational Media Department at Georgia State University. Lastly, I wish to thank Gaila Youtsey. Were it not for her word processing expertise, pages of the draft would still be in my typewriter.

—Robin J. Dixon

# The Patient Interview

*Chapter One*

## THE PATIENT INTERVIEW

Interviewing is one of the most important techniques available to the clinician in evaluating the respiratory patient. A careful and thoughtful patient interview can be a valuable tool in arriving at or eliminating a diagnosis. A hurried or superficial interview may be useless or, worse, misleading to someone following the patient. Like a child's first steps, one's first interviews will undoubtedly be awkward; however, with practice, interviewing the patient will become easier, and one should feel more comfortable.

The interview is considered by many clinicians to be the cornerstone of clinical medicine. Unfortunately, it is often neglected in the student's training, and many instructors are not skilled in the appropriate technique. In such cases, a most valuable clinical skill is not passed on to the student.

It is important to realize that the interview is not merely a series of stereotyped questions to be asked in a perfunctory manner. Some areas should be delved into more deeply, while other areas may be sufficiently covered with a single question. The depth of questioning that is appropriate often depends on the individual patient's responses and the clinical environment.

## Clinical Approach

The following section is designed to help the clinician obtain the optimum results from a patient interview by describing the proper approach to the patient, how to act toward the patient during the interview, and the types of questions which should be asked. It is also helpful for the beginning practitioner to know the characteristics of a poor interview; in this way, some of the potential pitfalls can be avoided. Finally, the categories that make for a complete history and what information the clinician should elicit in each category will be described.

### *Privacy*

In setting up the interview, try to obtain as much privacy as possible; preferably only the clinician and patient would be present. The presence of a third party might inhibit free discussion, and the observer may have somewhat distorted opinions. There may be situations in which a third person would be helpful, such as when the patient is mentally impaired or is a child. In these circumstances, the clinician *must* rely on another person for valuable information. Also, when arranging the interview, allow enough time to do a thorough job. If the interview is hurried, not only will the patient get a feeling that no one is interested in his problems, but also important areas are likely to be skipped or covered in a cursory manner.

### *Initiating the Interview*

The first thing one should do upon entering the patient's room is introduce oneself to the patient and explain one's reason for being there. When the patient has been referred for a consultation, it is helpful in establishing credibility if the name of the referring physician is used. For example: "Hello, Mrs. Jones. My name is Bill Smith. I am a therapist in the respiratory therapy department. Dr. Young has asked us to help him in evaluating your respiratory system..." The most awkward part of the interview is the very beginning because most people do not know how to begin a conversation with a stranger. Therefore, it is important for the practitioner, as well as the patient, to feel comfortable and relaxed. It will help to remember that most patients want someone to talk to and to listen to their problems. The clinician must be able to initiate the conversation effectively with the patient. In an effort to "break the ice", open the conversation with a few pleasantries to help the patient feel more at ease.

### *Attitude*

During the interview, the patient will, no doubt, be watching the clinician closely. One's appearance, dress, mannerisms, voice and attitude all contribute to the patient's trust. Your attitude and reaction to the patient's problems will create a greater impression than your knowledge and skills.

There is no substitute for interest on the part of the clinician. If the patient senses an attitude of sincerity and warmth, he is more likely to freely relate any health problems. There is, however, a difference between being friendly and being overly familiar; unless one knows the patient personally, no first names should be used. It is equally important to maintain a professional relationship with the patient.

A professional attitude is difficult to describe. Part of this attitude comes from characteristics of one's personality: honesty, strength of character, maturity, and gentleness. Other aspects contributing to professionalism, such as good judgement and discretion, are learned.

Having a professional attitude also means knowing how to deal with the uncooperative patient. This will require patience, understanding, and remembering that the patient is *ill*. Illness often causes a person to act out of character, and sometimes this is manifested as resentment. The sick patient may resent authority. Maintenance of a good sense of humor and a positive attitude may relieve some of the patient's resentment.

When talking with the patient, it is important to remember that the patient is an individual with unique problems and anxieties. In the early stages of the patient's care plan, the patient may be uninformed about his health status; this ignorance may enhance the patient's fears. If the patient is given reassurance that the staff is concerned about the individual as well as the disease process, this will go a long way toward building confidence and trust and allaying these fears. An important way in which reassurance is provided in a nonverbal manner is by remaining calm, since anxiety is often contagious.

Patients have within themselves a feeling of self-acceptance and a desire to be accepted by others. Sometimes divulging information that exposes the patient's weaknesses conflicts with the clinician's efforts to maintain this feeling of acceptance. The patient's vulnerability in such a case can interfere with his or her ability to share important personal information with the clinician.

Being empathetic can help the interviewer to gain the patient's confidence and encourages the patient to express personal feelings without embarrassment. This involves recognizing and accepting the patient's feelings and his expression of these feelings without criticism. Empathy does not involve giving advice or reassurance concerning the patient's illness. If a patient says: "I really thought I would be able to walk to the mailbox by now without getting short of breath", an appropriate response would be: "When you can't walk as far as you used to, I can see how you might get discouraged." This statement allows for self-expression without interjecting personal opinion or closing the topic.

## Proper Questioning Techniques

Students learning the art of interviewing often wonder what questions to ask their patients. For the first several interviews, it is suggested that the student follow an outline at the bedside. One should not feel embarrassed to use an outline until the mechanics of history-taking have been appropriately developed. Use an outline as a guide, then use experience in following up on a line of questioning. The student will discover that, as more histories are taken, history-taking becomes easier until it is second nature. Also, it is very helpful to observe others as they obtain a history. By observing, one can learn some effective questions and style differences which can be incorporated into the next interview.

Since the interview is a means of communication, it should be relaxed, frank and open, flexible and clear. The physical setting should be comfortable and free of interruption, and the conversation should be smooth and free of uncomfortable pauses. Even though the interview is formalized, it should not be stiff or rigid. The patient is simply seeking a service which is not available from his family or friends, and the interview is simply a conversation with a particular purpose in which respective roles have been set to that end.

After having exchanged a few pleasantries with the patient, do not begin the actual interview with questions such as, "What brought you here?" or "What's wrong with you?"; these are things which the patient wants you to tell him, eventually. The goal at this point is to have the patient tell his own story in his own way. A better way of opening the interview is with a question such as, "Tell me about your troubles" or "What seems to be the problem?". This approach gets the patient to relate his own reason(s) for seeking medical attention.

During the interview, speak in a clear, soft tone of voice. Even if an outline is followed, the questions should not be read to the patient in a monotone voice. Try to become familiar with the outline prior to seeing the patient, so that the interview flows smoothly.

A good interview requires structure and direction, and one of the most efficient ways to direct the interview is to phrase the questions properly. Proper phrasing of questions elicits the relevant information efficiently and in an unbiased fashion. There are several types of questions the interviewer can use to elicit the most informative and undistorted responses.

Since the object of the medical history is to lead the patient through an account of his illness in an unbiased way, care must be taken to avoid suggestive questions. Therefore, the *open-ended* or *neutral question* should be used whenever possible. This type of question is structured so as not to suggest a particular response by the patient. "Tell me about your shortness of breath" is an open-ended or neutral question; such a question encourages a statement in the patient's own words. Even a short question such as, "What do you mean?" accomplishes the same goal.

Whenever the patient has difficulty remembering certain facts, the *direct question* can be used. A direct question requires a specific (often yes or no type) answer. This type of question is efficient and helps to prevent the patient from digressing to irrelevant topics. "Does your chest hurt when you cough?" is a direct question. Though direct questions are efficient and to the point, this type of question should be used in moderation since too many of these questions may overwhelm the patient. Additionally, one must be careful not to put words into the patient's mouth. And it is important to remember that some patients will answer "yes" to almost all questions regardless of whether or not this is the correct answer; others will answer "no" to almost all questions. To avoid this, try rewording the question in the opposite manner. For example, if one wants to know whether sitting up in bed facilitates breathing for the patient who habitually answers "no" after asking exactly that, ask "Does lying down make it easier for you to breathe?". If the patient's answer is something like, "That's when it's hard to breathe," this answer is probably correct.

Many patients hesitate in their responses because they are not sure how much information is necessary about certain topics. Statements such as, "Anything else?" or "And then what?" stimulate the patient to continue. In many instances, a simple nod of the head is enough to encourage the patient to proceed.

With interviewing experience one discovers that the most fruitful interviews result from using all the types of questions. An open-ended question can be used to begin discussion on a topic, supplementary statements encourage the patient to continue, and a direct question can be posed to probe for a more informative answer when a response is inadequate. Table 1-1 lists the different types of questions used in interviews with examples of each.

**Table 1-1. Types of questions used in interviews and examples.**

| Open-ended or neutral question | Direct question | Supplementary statement |
|---|---|---|
| "What seems to be the problem?" | "Do you get dizzy often?" | "Anything else?" |
| "Tell me about your shortness of breath." | "How long have you noticed this fatigue?" | "I see." |
| "What do you mean?" | "Do you cough more in the morning?" | "Is that right?" |
| "Can you describe the sensation in your chest?" | "How much sputum do you cough up?" | "And then what?" |

Finally, make sure when asking questions that the patient understands *exactly* what is being asked. Try to evaluate the patient's educational background and use terminology that the patient will understand. This will probably necessitate using similes and layman's terms. For example, it will probably be more meaningful to the patient to ask, "Do you cough up blood?" than to ask "Do you experience hemoptysis?". Likewise, make sure that what the patient says is what the patient means. For example, the patient may admit to coughing up blood, but further inquiry may reveal that the patient is *vomiting* blood. For an interview to be effective the patient must understand the interviewer's questions and the interviewer must understand the patient's answers.

## *Nonverbal Communication*

In addition to using different questioning techniques, certain forms of nonverbal communication are helpful in achieving maximum results in an interview. When talking with the patient, maintain eye contact. This not only establishes a nonverbal line of communication but also helps maintain interviewer concentration on the patient's responses. It also minimizes the patient's tendency to ramble. On the other hand, do not stare at the patient, as this tends to make the patient self-conscious, especially if the patient is shy. It is also helpful to watch the patient's facial expressions during the interview, as these can be quite informative. The patient's facial expression can tip-off the clinician about a sensitive subject or even help the clinician determine whether the question is understood.

## Listening

Good interviewer listening habits are also critical to a successful patient interview. Intelligent listening is an art in itself; much important information concerning the patient and his problems can be gained in no other way. Patients want to tell their problems to someone, and they may volunteer information that is difficult to elicit through questioning if they feel that the interviewer is listening carefully. Careful listening is an important way in which the clinician can demonstrate his concern for the patient and his problems and thereby win the patient's confidence.

During the interview, patients may reveal some unexpected facts concerning their problems. While it is important to show concern for these problems and the patient, do not show overconcern or blatant surprise at a response. Patients are quick to pick up on staff reactions, and a show of surprise may inhibit them from volunteering important parts of their medical history. If a sensitive subject is brought up and the patient begins to cry, it is best to remain quiet momentarily. Typically, the patient will regain his composure and proceed to apologize. It is at this time that the interviewer should say some words of reassurance. The patient may be just now accepting the fact that he has a serious problem, and willingness to be there and listen can be comforting to the patient. After a moment, the interview may be continued.

When listening, it is important to determine the patient's reliability as a source of information. If the patient is unduly stressed, afraid or anxious, he may exaggerate his answers and thereby provide a misleading history. The patient may also be under the influence of certain medications which alter the mental status (e.g., analgesics).

Once the patient begins answering a question, try to avoid unnecessary interruptions. Constantly breaking into the patient's response not only sidetracks the patient but also makes putting information in chronological order difficult. If more specific questions are necessary to clarify the patient's response, these may be asked after the patient is finished answering the initial question.

## Potential Pitfalls

A medical history may be inadequate for various reasons, most of which can be attributed to interviewer technique. Extensive research has been performed on why some interviews are less satisfactory (Barbee, 1967), and awareness of these potential pitfalls will help one to avoid them. Table 1-2 identifies the overall characteristics of a good interview.

Some interviews are inadequate because of errors in data collection. In some instances the clinician fails to ask the patient important questions, such as completely omitting questions pertaining to any previous lung disease. Another common error is failure to record significant negative responses by the patient; in some cases these can be as important as positive answers. For example, the patient may admit to wheezing, but the clinician fails to record the fact that the patient has no known allergies.

Another reason for poor interviews involves the structure of the interview. Some clinicians do not try to put the patient at ease in the beginning and immediately begin asking delicate questions. The patient is already apprehensive about relating personal information, so a warming-up period should precede serious questioning. Also, an interview is not properly structured if one needlessly repeats questions because of a failure to record the patient's responses. Information obtained in the interview is part of the patient's medical record, so all of the patient's responses should be recorded. Another commonly made structuring error is jumping between unrelated areas. When inquiring about the

10

**Table 1-2. Characteristics of a good interview.**

---

*Privacy*

---

Preferably, only clinician and patient will be present; a third party may inhibit discussion.

Allow enough time for a thorough patient history.

*Interviewer Attitude*

---

Maintain a positive and professional attitude.

Show interest, empathy, and acceptance of the patient.

Show concern with the patient as an individual.

*Proper Questioning Technique*

---

Use neutral or open-ended questions to begin the interview and allow the patient to tell his or her own story.

Use supplementary statements to encourage the hesitant patient to continue.

Use direct questions when a more specific and informative answer is required.

Make sure that the patient understands the questions.

*Nonverbal Communication*

---

Maintain eye contact with the patient, but do not stare intently at them.

Watch the patient's facial expressions, which can be quite informative.

*Listening*

---

Listen carefully to what the patient has to say.

Do not show overconcern or blatant surprise at a patient's response.

Determine the patient's reliability as a source of information.

Avoid unnecessary interruptions while the patient is talking.

---

patient's allergic reaction to certain medications, do not begin asking questions about the smoking history of the patient only to return to the topic of allergies. A well-organized interview can be both accurate and time-saving.

Attitude can be responsible for an unproductive interview. If the clinician seems preoccupied or not interested in the patient's problems, the patient senses this and will probably be less willing to confide in the clinician. In addition, if the interviewer acts too friendly or not friendly enough, this can negatively affect the rapport between the interviewer and the patient and make information-gathering more difficult. If the patient senses an overly informal attitude, it might be difficult for the patient to take the interview seriously. It is also difficult to have an effective interview when there is a lack of patient eye contact. As mentioned above, this can result in the patient digressing to irrelevant topics.

Other errors commonly made in interviews are those in communication. If the interviewer constantly interrupts, not allowing the patient to complete his responses, important facts may be omitted from the history. Misleading information may result from asking too many suggestive questions; in some cases this amounts to putting words in the patient's mouth, as some patients will agree to whatever is suggested. Additionally, the patient can be overcome by too many direct questions, which are usually answered with only a "yes" or "no". Asking this kind of question prevents the patient from giving supportive information. Finally, inaccurate interviews can be attributed to the interviewer's using medical jargon not understood by the patient. Patients rarely admit to not understanding a question; instead, they tend to agree with whatever is being asked, which results in misinformation. Table 1-3 summarizes the common errors leading to poor interviews.

In order to achieve maximum results and accurate information in a medical interview, remember that the patient is a person. Work at establishing a mutual trust with the patient. Utilize different types of questions and lead the patient through the medical history in an organized manner. After several interviews, one will have discovered what questions work best in a given situation. Now that the mechanics of the interview have been discussed, attention will be directed toward the content areas which should be covered with the patient in a medical history.

**Table 1-3. Common errors leading to poor interviews.**

### *Errors in Data Collection*

Interviewer failed to ask important questions.

Interviewer failed to follow-up important leads.

Interviewer's omission of important negative responses by patient.

### *Poor Structuring of Interview*

Failure to put patient at ease.

Interviewer's repetition of questions.

Interviewer's failure to record patient responses.

Interviewer jumped back and forth between unrelated areas.

### *Errors in Attitude*

Interviewer seemed preoccupied, not interested.

Interviewer acted overly friendly or not friendly enough.

Lack of eye contact with patient.

Interviewer interjected his personal feelings into interview.

### *Errors in Communication*

Interviewer continually interrupted the patient's responses.

Interviewer put words in patient's mouth by asking too many suggestive questions.

Interviewer asked too many direct questions, thereby preventing the patient from giving supportive information.

Interviewer used medical jargon.

# The Patient History

*Chapter Two*

## THE PATIENT HISTORY

### Chief Complaint

The chief complaint is a short statement in the patient's own words describing the main problem for which the patient has sought medical attention. The idea is to obtain a spontaneous statement from the patient about the main problem with minimal guidance. A good guideline is that the patient should say more than the interviewer. The chief complaint may be something like: "shortness of breath" or "pain in the chest." At this point, most patients wait for the clinician to indicate how they should proceed. This is the time to utilize a questioning technique that encourages the patient to continue, such as, "Is anything else bothering you?" or even a nod of the head. It is also useful to get the patient to recount the symptoms several times because new information is disclosed each time. Characteristics of the symptom, however, should not be dealt with in this section but should be included in the history of the present illness. Again, note the symptom or symptoms that bother the patient the most.

The chief complaint is recorded in the patient's own words and not in terms such as "dyspnea or exertion" or "angina pectoris." Some patients may complain of having "emphysema;" although this may very well be true, you should not accept the patient's diagnosis. During the course of the interview, the symptoms which led to the patient's diagnosis should be identified. It is important that the interviewer not jump on the initial problem stated by the patient and begin asking direct questions; doing so doesn't give the patient an opportunity to mention and describe other problems associated with the chief complaint. The goal is to get the patient to relate *all* the problems.

### History of Present Illness

When obtaining the history of the present illness, allow patients to tell their own story in their own words. If the patient starts to ramble on, you may need to keep the story in line by skillfully directing the interview. The history of the patient's present illness should be a well-organized elaboration of the chief complaint(s)—a chronological history of each symptom about which the patient complains.

During the course of the interview it will become evident which symptoms belong with the present illness and which symptoms relate to other problems. The most difficult situations are those in which the symptoms reflect more than one disease, such as pneumonia in a patient with chronic bronchitis.

To aid in the diagnostic process, each symptom, as it relates to the present illness, is characterized in terms of the following: date of onset, nature of the complaint, course of the complaint, location, exacerbations, and treatment. It is suggested that these characteristics be memorized because they are the basis for the questions to be asked about each symptom.

### Date of Onset

Whenever possible, the clinician should elicit from the patient the specific date each symptom began. It is acceptable to use a date of reference such as the hospital admission date to indicate when a symptom was first noticed: "The patient first noticed chest pain three weeks prior to admission (3/5/82)", for example. It is best to avoid terms such as "last week" unless they can be related to a specific date; such information will be meaningless when reviewing the medical record at a later date.

The duration of each symptom also conveys important information regarding a disease process. It should be established whether a symptom lasts for minutes, hours, days, weeks, or months. For example, a productive cough for several days may be indicative of an upper respiratory infection, whereas a productive cough for several months of the year may be a clue to chronic bronchitis.

### Nature of Complaint

It is important to note the character of the discomfort about which the patient complains. Often it is difficult for the patient to describe the sensation felt, so it is helpful to suggest descriptive terms like burning, aching, sharp, dull, or throbbing. Also, the severity of the discomfort should be noted: is it mild, moderate, or severe? Usually a discomfort can be described by a word. In cases where the patient uses multiple adjectives to describe a sensation, detailed questioning may be necessary to determine the exact nature of the complaint.

### Course of Complaint

Besides knowing when each symptom began, it is equally important to determine the evolution of each symptom. How has the symptom progressed from the time it was first noticed until the present? Also, it should be determined whether there are any particular activities associated with changes in a symptom. For example: Does the symptom change when the patient stands up or lies down? Does the patient notice any change in the symptom with exercise? It is important to record what the patient associates with change in a symptom, no matter how mundane; sometimes eating certain foods can precipitate wheezing, for example. Also, the interviewer should ascertain the progress of the symptom in terms of its severity: has the shortness of breath gotten worse or better since it was first noticed?

### Location

If the patient complains of pain or discomfort in the chest, a specific location should be established. A response such as, "pain in my side" is unacceptable. Ask the patient to point specifically to where the pain is most intense. Also, determine whether the discomfort is localized or radiates to other areas. If the patient points to the sternum and says the pain is there, it is important to determine whether the sensation experienced is actually pain or another discomfort; commonly, substernal "pain" is more of a tightness or heavy feeling in the chest. When recording the location of the pain or discomfort, use permanent, immobile structures as reference points. "2 centimeters right of the left nipple" would be an inadequate description because the nipple will move in women with pendulous breasts (and even in some men). The location of the pain or discomfort should be described in such a way that anyone following your description would be able to find the lesion or point of discomfort.

### Exacerbations

Many diseases are characterized by exacerbations and remissions during their course. There might be seasonal changes or even a daily change in the severity of the disorder, and this should be noted. For example, patients with byssinosis characteristically complain of fever and dyspnea on Mondays which disappear as the week progresses. This is due to a tolerance quickly built up during the week, and the fever only reappears after an absence from exposure to cotton (Kleinerman, 1974). Also, extrinsic asthmatics may complain more of wheezing in the spring when the pollen season is at its peak.

### Treatment

What, if anything, has been done to alleviate a symptom? If the patient is presently on any medications for the symptom, the name, dosage, and frequency of each medication should be recorded. Some patients will try home remedies, and these, too, should be recorded. Perhaps the symptom disappeared as a result of taking measures to alleviate it only to spontaneously return; if so, this, too, should be recorded in the patient's history.

By this point in the interview the clinician should know why the patient is seeking medical attention and have a description and chronological history of each symptom. This description and history of the present illness should include information on when each symptom was first noticed, the duration of each symptom, the characteristics of each symptom, the progress of each symptom, any activities associated with changes in a symptom, the exact location of each symptom, and past and present treatment of each symptom. If treatment was administered, the name, dosage, and frequency of medication should be noted. Table 2-1 outlines the topics included in an organized history of the present illness. Once the clinician has this information, background information on the patient's past medical history, his family's medical history, and his personal history should be obtained.

## Past Medical History

The purpose of constructing the past medical history is to determine the past health of the patient, including illnesses,

## Table 2-1. Guideline for the history of present illness.

### Date of Onset

Record the specific date each symptom began and the duration of each symptom.

### Nature of Complaint

Note the character of each discomfort (burning, aching, sharp, dull, throbbing, etc.) and the severity of each discomfort (mild, moderate, or severe). Usually a discomfort can be described by a single word.

### Course of Complaint

How has the symptom changed since it was first noticed?

Are there any specific activities associated with changes in the symptom (does the symptom change when the patient stands up or lies down?)?

Note the progress of each symptom in terms of its severity (has the shortness of breath gotten worse or better since it was first noticed?).

### Location

Determine the specific location of each discomfort.

Is the discomfort localized or does it radiate?

Determine whether the sensation experienced is actually pain or another discomfort (e.g., what is commonly called substernal "pain" is often more of a tightness or heavy feeling in the chest).

Use permanent, immobile structures as reference points when recording the location of the pain or discomfort.

### Exacerbations

Are there daily or seasonal changes in the severity of the disorder?

### Treatment

What has been done to alleviate the symptom?

Note the results of any treatment measures (home remedies or professional treatment).

Record the name, dosage, and frequency of each medication the patient is currently taking for relief of the symptom.

previous hospitalizations, accidents, and allergies. This is an important part of the interview because it can yield information concerning the etiology of the present illness. It has been shown (Lebowitz, 1977) that the past medical history is a strong predictor of current medical problems, so an organized approach to the previous medical history is important. It's hard for most patients to remember, in chronological sequence, all their medical problems over a period of many years. Therefore, as opposed to the method of questioning used in the history of the present illness, direct questions have been shown to be most effective in getting an accurate past medical history.

Begin the past medical history with a brief summary of the past health status of the patient, which should be described as either "good," "average," or "poor". Record the date and findings of the patient's last physical exam. If past records are required, it is also helpful to know who performed each exam.

### Childhood Diseases

Next, inquire about any childhood or infectious diseases in the patient's past. First, ask the patient if he or she actually contracted or was just exposed to measles, mumps, chicken pox, tonsillitis, or any socially communicable diseases. Concerning a pulmonary history, ask if the patient had any lung trouble before the age of sixteen. Also ask if the patient ever had any of the more common pulmonary disorders: attacks of bronchitis, pneumonia, chronic bronchitis, emphysema, hay fever, or asthma. The presence of any allergies or hypersensitivity reactions to foods, drugs, or environmental conditions should also be determined. If the patient responds affirmatively to any of these queries, several follow-up questions should be asked: "Was it confirmed by a doctor?" and "At what age did you first have it?" Many patients who claim they had a "touch of bronchitis" actually did not. No diagnosis made by a patient should be accepted at face value. After this initial survey, determine whether the patient had any other chest-related illnesses, chest injuries, or chest operations, and if so, record what they were.

### Previous Hospitalizations

As part of the patient's past medical history, previous hospitalizations and surgical procedures should be recorded.

Record the dates of all previous hospitalizations and the reasons for admission. If the patient has undergone surgery, record the type of surgery, the date, and any complications associated with the surgical procedure or the anesthesia.

## Accidents

Any serious injuries resulting in fractures or unconsciousness should be recorded. Injuries such as minor burns or abrasions can be omitted from the history since these usually do not warrant medical attention. Any penetrating wounds or complications from minor injuries, however, should be entered into the patient's record. For example, the patient may have contracted tetanus after having stepped on a nail.

## Illnesses

Since many people in our society suffer from heart trouble and/or hypertension, a complete past medical history should include inquiry into these areas. If the patient responds affirmatively to the question, "Has a doctor ever told you that you have heart trouble or high blood pressure?" ask whether the patient has required any treatment for either condition and what that treatment included. This will give the interviewer a clue as to the severity of either illness.

Sometimes patients will forget about past illnesses; inquiring whether the patient has ever been put on antibiotics can help to uncover some forgotten illnesses, as having undergone such therapy indicates the presence of an infection in the patient's past. Not uncommonly has a forgotten past case of pneumonia been discovered after questioning about previous antibiotic therapy. A patient may not think it important to mention that he has been placed on prophylactic antibiotic therapy prior to dental work, yet if such a scenario emerges the clinician should suspect the potential presence of mitral valve disease or subacute bacterial endocarditis.

## Family History

The patient may want to know why it is important for the clinician to collect information on his family's medical history. The clinician should explain that some diseases, such as diabetes mellitus, hypertension, cystic fibrosis, and allergies can "run in the family." Also, the family history pro-vides information concerning the patient's chances of contracting diseases such as emphysema.

Begin the family history by determining the age and health status of both natural parents. If a parent is deceased, the age at which the parent died and the cause of death should be recorded. Inquire whether either of the parents was told by a doctor that he or she had a chronic lung condition such as chronic bronchitis, emphysema, asthma, lung cancer, or other chest conditions. Next, determine the age and cause of death of any deceased blood-line relatives. Questions concerning the health status of grandparents and siblings should be included; exposure to tuberculosis has been uncovered after it was discovered that a child had visited infected grandparents. Finally, ask the patient if there have been any incidences of allergy, kidney disease, or nervous or mental disorder in the family.

## Personal History

The purpose of taking the personal history is to provide information about the general characteristics of the patient. It is helpful to know what the patient's reactions are to his or her environment, work, family, and friends. More specifi-cally, the personal history of the patient should include answers to questions concerning place of birth and place(s) of residence, socioeconomic status, occupational history, educational background, habits, and any medications the patient is taking.

## Life History

A *brief* description of the patient's life history is appro-priate for the medical record. Information on the patient's place of birth and his or her past and present residences is all that should be included in this part of the patient's medical record. This information is important because certain pulmonary diseases, such as some of the pneumoconioses, are peculiar to specific regions of the country. For example, histoplasmosis is endemic to the Ohio and Mississippi River valleys. If the patient spent time in a foreign country while in the armed services, for example, this also might point to a certain disease. The clinician should inquire whether the patient spent any time in third world countries because of the potential for contracting parasitic diseases in these locations.

## Socioeconomic Status

Questions in this area are designed to determine the patient's state of social adjustment and help the clinician interpret any organic disease in light of emotional tendencies. Questions are directed toward the patient's business life, work habits, and financial status. Is the patient mature in his approach to his medical problems? What are the patient's living conditions like? In some asthmatics, an attack can be precipitated by emotional stress or environmental factors such as dust or house pets. Inquiry into this area provides the clinician information regarding the possible causes of the asthmatic attacks.

## Occupational History

It is generally recognized that certain occupations are directly related to the incidence of pulmonary disease. Therefore, all past and present jobs should be recorded in the patient's history. The interviewer should inquire about exposures to noxious gases, fumes, or other irritating substances such as dust. Perhaps the patient worked with some wild or domestic animals. There are some occupations which, on the surface, are not obviously related to pulmonary disorders. For example, the patient states that he has worked in the brake-lining business for twelve years. Though this may appear to be a benign occupation, brake linings contain asbestos, and such an occupation could lead to asbestosis. Other occupational pulmonary diseases and their causes and symptoms are listed in Table 2-2.

## Education

Determine the educational level of the patient. Knowing this background helps the clincian direct the interview toward the patient's level of understanding. The responses of a highly educated person tend to be more reliable than those of a patient with only a primary school education.

## Medications

By this stage of the interview, the clinician should be aware of any medications the patient has taken for treat-

**Table 2-2. Etiologies and symptoms of occupational pulmonary diseases.**

| Condition | Etiology | Primary complaint(s) |
|---|---|---|
| asbestosis | asbestos | dyspnea on exertion |
| bagassosis | sugar cane | fever, dyspnea |
| byssinosis | cotton, hemp | "Monday fever" |
| coal worker's pneumoconiosis | coal | nonproductive cough |
| farmer's lung | moulded hay | fever, dyspnea |
| maple bark disease | fungus in maple bark | dyspnea on exertion |
| mushroom worker's disease | mushroom compost | dyspnea |
| ornithosis | dry excreta from birds | fever, cough |
| sequoiosis | moulded redwood sawdust | fever, malaise |
| silicosis | silica or silicon dioxide | dyspnea on exertion |
| suberosis | moulded oak bark, cork dust | fever, nonproductive cough |

ment of the chief complaint(s). The clinician should determine whether the patient has taken medications for any other reasons as well. This is particularly true for any over-the-counter medications, which can easily be overlooked. Knowing what these medications are can provide information about systemic problems other than the chief complaint and should prompt further questioning regarding the reason for these medications. Again, the name of the drug, dosage, frequency, and length of time taken should be recorded in the patient's history.

## Personal Habits

Personal habits of the patient include those related to sleeping, eating, exercise, alcohol, and smoking. Does the patient eat a balanced diet? How much coffee does the patient drink? Does the patient drink alcohol and, if so, what type and how much does the patient drink? Avoid using terms such as "moderate drinker" or "excessive smoker". Not only are these descriptions inexact, but using them is making a value judgement. What is excessive to one person may be moderate to another. The patient's level of consumption of tobacco or alcohol should be recorded in number of cigarettes smoked per day or number of drinks per day. If the patient is or was a tobacco user, a more specific smoking history should be obtained.

## Smoking History

Tobacco smoking, which includes cigarette, pipe, and cigar smoking, is associated with an increased morbidity and mortality in various diseases. Among these are carcinoma (mouth, larynx, lung, and bladder), chronic bronchitis, emphysema, and coronary artery disease. A cigarette smoker is defined as a person who has smoked at least twenty packs of cigarettes or at least one cigarette per day for at least one year in a lifetime (Ferris, 1978). Many patients admit to smoking less than they actually do, partly because of the attitudes of non-smokers toward smokers and also because the patient fears what the clinician will think. So rather than asking the patient, "Do you smoke cigarettes?", begin by asking if the patient has *ever* smoked cigarettes. Having admitted to past smoking habits may make the patient less reluctant to admit to present tobacco use. If the patient has smoked cigarettes in the past, determine if smoking still continues. Follow-up questions should include "How old were you when you first began regular smoking?" and, if the patient has stopped smoking completely, "How old were you when you stopped?". This is important because the cessation of smoking is associated with a decrease in morbidity (Francis, 1976). Also, inquire about the number of cigarettes presently smoked each day and the average number of cigarettes smoked per day during the entire time the patient has used tobacco. Cigarette smoking is usually quantitated in pack-years. The number of pack-years equals the average number of packs smoked each day multiplied by the number of years of smoking. For example, a 20 pack-year history implies 1 pack per day for 20 years or 2 packs per day for 10 years, etc. Finally, ask the patient, "Do or did you ever inhale the smoke?". An affirmative response to this question might suggest more involved lung disease.

One should also inquire whether the patient has ever smoked a pipe. The same questions regarding cigarette use should be asked about pipe smoking; however, rather than asking about the number of "pipefuls" of tobacco smoked each week, record the number of ounces smoked per week. (A standard pouch contains 1 1/2 ounces.)

Finally, regarding tobacco use, determine whether the patient has ever smoked cigars. ("Yes" means more than one cigar per week for a year.) Again, the same questions mentioned above should be asked of the patient regarding cigar smoking, including whether or not the patient inhales the smoke.

At this juncture in the interview, the clinician should have a thorough understanding of the medical history of the patient. As one can tell, some parts of the history can be covered quickly, while others may require meticulous and detailed questioning, depending, of course, on the patient. There are, however, some very common symptoms of pulmonary disease about which the patient should be questioned, namely cough, phlegm, hemoptysis, dyspnea, orthopnea, chest pain, and wheezing. Because of their importance and characteristic association with pulmonary disease, a detailed description of and the questions which should be asked concerning each of these symptoms have been reserved for a separate chapter.

# Cardiopulmonary
# Symptoms

*Chapter Three*

## CARDIOPULMONARY SYMPTOMS

As generally employed, the term *symptom* refers to any perceptible change in the body or its functions that is indicative of disease. This chapter is concerned primarily with symptoms of cardiopulmonary origin such as cough, sputum, hemoptysis, dyspnea, chest pain, and wheezing.

The purpose of evaluating the history carefully and the physical findings systematically is to determine the pathophysiological processes involved in a disorder and thereby arrive at a diagnosis. Symptoms are often present before laboratory tests are useful in detecting a disorder. For this reason, and because a thorough history can often lead the clinician to the correct conclusion more readily than other diagnostic methods, one should never neglect an accurate and detailed history of the symptom(s).

## Cough

A cough is an expiratory blast of air occurring against a closed glottis. This may occur voluntarily or involuntarily via reflex stimulation. The involuntary cough is induced by stimulation of the glossopharyngeal nerve endings in the pharynx and afferent nerve endings of the vagus in the larynx, trachea, and large bronchi. A cough is basically a protective airway mechanism intended to clear the airway of mucus or any other foreign debris.

### Cough Mechanism

The cough mechanism can be divided into three distinct phases. First, in the inspiratory phase, air is drawn into the lungs prior to the cough. In the second, the compressive phase of cough, the thoracic, accessory, and abdominal muscles contract with a closed glottis, thereby building up intraabdominal and intrathoracic pressures. The transpulmonary pressures generated during a cough may be as high as 200 mm Hg; pressures of this magnitude can produce an expiratory flowrate exceeding 500 l/min. (Francis, 1976). In the third phase of cough, the expulsive phase, the glottis opens and the diaphragm pushes upward producing a rapid movement of air from the lower to the upper airways. The efficiency of a cough is directly related to the volume of air inspired prior to the cough and the velocity of the air flow during expulsion.

## Pulmonary Disease

Cough is one of the most common symptoms of pulmonary disease, and since a chronic or persistent cough is not part of the ordinary respiratory cycle it should always be considered abnormal. Obtaining an accurate history of cough is often difficult because 1) many patients swallow the sputum, 2) some patients underestimate the actual frequency of the cough, and 3) cigarette smokers tend to minimize symptoms related to their smoking. Questioning a family member of the patient is often more helpful in determining the actual frequency and severity of the cough.

Begin by asking the patient, "Do you usually have a cough?". Count a cough with the first smoke or on first going outside, and exclude clearing of the throat. If the patient responds in the affirmative, ask whether the patient usually coughs as much as four to six times a day, four or more days out of the week. This will help the interviewer determine how chronic the cough really is. Regardless of the patient's response, next ask whether the patient usually coughs at all, especially upon getting up. Also ask whether the patient coughs at all during the rest of the day or night. In order for the clinician to determine whether the cough is chronic, if any of the responses to the above questions is "yes" ask, "Do you usually cough like this on most days for three or more consecutive months during the course of a year?" and "How many years have you had this cough?". If a cough is present, determine the time of onset and the progress of the cough. Has the cough worsened or improved? Is the cough generally present in the morning only? Is the cough related to the patient's position? Is the cough seasonal? These questions should provide information concerning the characteristics and the severity of the cough. Table 3-1 lists the characteristics of the coughs associated with some of the common conditions in which cough is found.

**Table 3-1. Characteristics of cough in common conditions.**

| Condition | Characteristics of Cough |
|---|---|
| Acute infections | Paroxysmal day and night, without sputum |
| Asthma | Hacking, often wheezing, sometimes severe and persistent; often seasonal |
| Chronic bronchitis | Initially dry, becoming productive, worse in the morning |
| Bronchogenic carcinoma | Changes from usual cough; sometimes less productive, more severe or change in sound |
| Bronchial irritation | Continuing dry cough |
| Congestive heart failure | Intermittent, productive and associated with dyspnea and orthopnea, often nocturnal |

## Sputum

A discussion of cough is incomplete without a consideration of sputum. Mucus is produced by the goblet cells and the submucosal glands, both of which line the respiratory epithelium. Normal mucus is about 95% water; the other 5% is composed of protein, carbohydrate, DNA, cellular debris, and foreign substances. There is a gradual decrease in the water content of mucus from the epithelial surface to the luminal surface. Because of this, mucus has been divided into two layers: the more viscous gel layer and the sol layer, which is adjacent to the epithelial surface (see *Figure 3-1*).

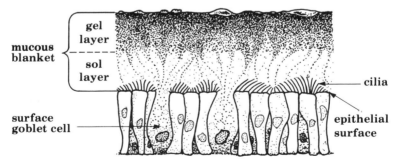

*Figure 3-1.* Backward movement of the cilia occurs entirely within the sol layer, while forward motion extends the cilia into the gel layer thereby moving the mucus toward the large airways.

33

### *Sputum Production*

A sheet of mucus (mucous blanket) (*Figure 3-1*) lines the respiratory tract from the glottis down to and including the respiratory bronchioles (Mitchell, 1970). The exact quantity of respiratory secretions in the healthy adult is uncertain but is estimated to be as much as 100 ml/day. This efficient transit of mucus is the primary factor in clearing the airways of foreign elements and microorganisms.

Just as chronic cough is always abnormal, sputum production is always a sign of disease. Because patients find it aesthetically unpleasant, they dispose of sputum as quickly as possible and often minimize or deny producing sputum altogether. (The terms mucus, sputum and phlegm are different words representing the same substance. Because a patient might not understand the first two terms, "phlegm" is used in the questions.) If the patient admits to a productive cough, determine whether it comes from the chest or from clearing the throat. "Do you usually bring up phlegm from your chest?" (Count sputum with the first smoke or on first going out-of-doors. Count swallowed sputum, but exclude secretions from the nose.) If the patient answers "yes" ask, "Do you usually bring up phlegm like this as much as twice a day, four or more days out of the week?".

If the patient does not usually have sputum production, ask whether he brings up phlegm at all upon getting up. Many patients have a more productive cough just after arising because their secretions have been mobilized into the upper airways while lying in a recumbent position during sleep. Then ask the patient, "Do you usually bring up phlegm at all during the rest of the day or night?". If the patient answers "yes" to any of these questions ask him whether he produces sputum like this on most days for three or more consecutive months during the year and how long he has had trouble with phlegm.

After the presence of sputum production has been established, the quantity of the expectorated material and the duration of sputum production should be recorded. Since most patients are unfamiliar with milliliters, and the anxious patient may have difficulty quantitating accurately, it is recommended that the clinician request the patient to quantitate his sputum production in terms of "cupsfull' (one cup equals 250 ml). If a productive cough is "normal" for a particular patient, as is the case with smokers, ask whether there have been any episodes of increased cough and sputum production lasting three weeks or more during the year. Such episodes indicate the possibility of the presence of chronic bronchitis.

### Sputum Characteristics

Besides the quantity of sputum produced, it is important to determine the characteristics of the secretions. If possible, have the patient produce some sputum so that you can observe the color, consistency, and odor. Sputum, by itself, is rarely diagnostic; however, it can prompt further questioning and laboratory analysis. Some of the different types of sputum, their characteristics and the conditions in which they are found are listed in Table 3-2.

**Table 3-2. Characteristics and associated conditions of different types of sputum.**

| Sputum | Characteristics and associated conditions |
|---|---|
| purulent | thick; yellow and malodorous or green (green purulent sputum is indicative of infection); found in bronchiectasis and lung abscess |
| mucoid | sticky, translucent; gray or white; difficult to expectorate; found in bronchitis and pneumonia |
| mucopurulent | a combination of mucoid and purulent sputum; contains yellow or green pus; found in bacterial infection |
| pink, frothy | pink; watery and foamy; found in pulmonary edema |

(From Rarey, K.P., and Youtsey, J.W., *Respiratory Patient Care*. Englewood Cliffs: Prentice-Hall, 1981.)

## Hemoptysis

The specific color of the sputum should be ascertained as this may indicate whether or not bleeding is present. If bleeding is present the color will usually be either bright red (new or active bleeding), pink (blood mixed with sputum), or dark (rusty) red (old blood). The expectorated material may be frank blood or blood mixed with sputum and may or may not contain clots. The length of time that the patient has experienced hemoptysis (the coughing up of blood) should be recorded in hours, days, weeks, or months. Also ask whether the hemoptysis is associated with any particular activity-(ies) (coughing, exercise, and/or position). Usually hemoptysis occurs after coughing and can recur over several hours or several years.

Hemoptysis is an extremely important symptom of pulmonary disease. When the patient presents with hemoptysis, there is a very real possibility of pulmonary hemorrhage. Associated symptoms can often suggest the cause of the hemoptysis. Is this the only episode or is this a problem of recurrent hemoptysis? If the patient is relatively young and has a history of recurrent pulmonary infections involving hemoptysis, bronchiectasis is suggested. Pleuritic chest pain, dyspnea, and scant amounts of dark red blood in the sputum suggest pulmonary infarction. A smoker over 40 years old who suffers from a chronic cough which recurrently produces bright red sputum may have bronchogenic cancer.

Because of its potential danger, determining the cause of hemoptysis is of top priority. Hemoptysis can result from trauma, inflammation, aspiration of foreign bodies, neoplasms, or cardiovascular disorders.

### Trauma

Hemoptysis can result from the lungs having been punctured by a fractured rib, a knife, or a gunshot wound. Inhaling irritating fumes or smoke can traumatize the lungs and result in bleeding into the airways. The tracheobronchial tree can be lacerated by a blunt trauma such as a steering wheel. Severe coughing can lacerate the tracheal mucosa and cause hemoptysis.

### Inflammation

Hemoptysis can also result from inflammation in the lung. Many years ago, tuberculosis was the leading cause of hemoptysis (Pierce, 1970). Since this disease has come under control, however, other inflammatory lesions have replaced tuberculosis as the most frequent causes of hemoptysis. Patients with pneumococcal pneumonia, for example, characteristically expectorate blood-tinged sputum. Necrotizing pneumonias such as those caused by Klebsiella and other gram negative organisms are also responsible for hemoptysis.

Fungal infections of the respiratory tract can cause cavitation or necrosis and result in bleeding into the airway. Hemoptysis can also result after the healing of a fungal infection from either a secondary bacterial infection or erosion of calcium deposits.

## Bronchiectasis

Hemoptysis is frequently seen in patients with saccular bronchiectasis. Because this disease involves destruction of the bronchi, patients who suffer from it are vulnerable to bacterial infections which may lead to mucosal ulcerations. In severe bronchiectasis, the bronchial arteries enlarge and hemorrhage from this blood supply can be severe.

## Aspiration of Foreign Bodies

Aspiration of foreign bodies can traumatize the airway mucosa and cause bleeding.

## Carcinoma

Bronchogenic carcinoma is the most common cause of hemoptysis in persons over the age of 45 (Kory, 1974; Pierce, 1970). Hemorrhage in bronchogenic cancer may be the result of mucosal ulceration or necrosis in the center of the tumor. Although hemoptysis is common in patients with bronchogenic carcinoma, it is rarely the presenting symptom. Other tumors, such as bronchial adenomas and hemangiomas, can also cause hemoptysis.

## Cardiovascular Disease

Cardiovascular conditions are another category to which hemoptysis can be attributed. Patients with pulmonary edema secondary to left ventricular failure characteristically expectorate pink, frothy sputum. Mitral stenosis is a common cause of hemoptysis, especially when there is severe pulmonary hypertension; however, hemoptysis usually occurs in the later stages of this disease, after the diagnosis has already been established. Another common vascular cause of hemoptysis is pulmonary embolism, especially when it results in pulmonary infarction. Typically, pulmonary infarction occurs in patients with preexisting cardiac disease and in hospitalized patients following surgery or an acute illness.

### Source of Hemoptysis

Hemoptysis, because it is such a frightening symptom, usually prompts the patient to seek medical attention. The presenting complaint is usually "spitting up blood," and since the bleeding often isn't present by the time the patient seeks medical help, a careful history is very necessary. It is most important to make sure that the blood did not originate in the nasal passages or oropharynx. It must also be established that the patient *coughed* up the blood and did not vomit it. Because patients are often frightened by blood, they may confuse coughing and vomiting. Once it has been established that the patient coughed up the material, ask whether the secretions consisted entirely of blood or the sputum was just spotted with blood.

The actual cause of hemoptysis often cannot be determined by the history, the physical exam, and the chest x-ray alone. Sometimes tomograms, bronchoscopy, and sputum cytology may be required, and even these studies fail to determine the cause of hemoptysis in about 15% of the patients with hemoptysis (Pursel, 1961).

## Dyspnea

Dyspnea, difficult or labored respiration, is one of the most common and, unfortunately, one of the most poorly understood symptoms of cardiopulmonary disease. The term "dyspnea" implies a subjective awareness on the part of the patient of having difficulty in breathing; it is the sensation experienced when the patient is conscious of an increased respiratory effort. Usually, the patient will say something like, "I'm short of breath" or "I can't catch my breath." The patient may complain of a "tightness" in the chest or fatigue while walking up the driveway. Due to the subjectivity of dyspnea, however, one should be sensitive to the patient's description.

### Cardiopulmonary Disease

Dyspnea is not always a symptom of disease. For example, it is completely normal for a person to be aware of respiratory effort after exercise. Dyspnea is a symptom of cardiac and/or pulmonary disease only when the patient experiences it when at rest or when it is inappropriate for the level of exercise. The patient may have been able to walk up two flights of stairs at a moderate pace without experiencing shortness of breath in the past, but in the last six months has noticed difficulty in climbing up one flight of stairs. It helps in evaluating dyspnea to compare present levels of exercise-induced dyspnea to past levels of exercise-induced dyspnea. The degree of dyspnea experienced will vary from patient to patient and depend upon age, body size, and the patient's state of physical conditioning.

Dyspnea can be the result of a variety of disturbances, either cardiac or pulmonary in origin: uneven ventilation in relation to blood flow, airway obstruction, decreased lung compliance, diffusion abnormalities, inadequate cardiac output, and right-to-left shunting. Although a great deal has been written about dyspnea, many physicians still have difficulty distinguishing pulmonary from cardiac dyspnea. A rapid onset of dyspnea is suggestive of a pulmonary embolism, pulmonary edema, acute bronchoconstriction, a spontaneous pneumothorax, or anxiety. Dyspnea resulting from left ventricular failure has a more gradual onset and worsens without treatment; this kind of dypsnea is also associated with paroxysmal nocturnal dyspnea and orthopnea. Dyspnea secondary to chronic obstructive pulmonary disease (COPD) is also gradual in onset and often gets worse in cold weather and during upper respiratory infections. In patients with both COPD and left ventricular failure, determination of the cause of dyspnea is more difficult since some of these patients become dyspneic in the supine position, which resembles the situation in orthopnea. Table 3-3 lists some of the cardiopulmonary causes of dyspnea.

### Inspiratory and Expiratory Dyspnea

Dyspnea can be either inspiratory or expiratory in nature. Inspiratory dyspnea usually results from obstruction of the upper airway due to tumors, laryngeal edema, foreign bodies, or vocal cord paralysis which inhibits the inward

**Table 3-3. Cardiopulmonary causes of dyspnea.**

| | |
|---|---|
| emphysema | croup |
| bronchitis | epiglottitis |
| asthma | congestive heart failure |
| cystic fibrosis | pulmonary edema |
| pulmonary fibrosis | pulmonary embolism |
| foreign body aspiration | spontaneous pneumothorax |
| vocal cord paralysis | kyphoscoliosis |
| tracheal tumors | neuromuscular disease |
| laryngeal edema | anxiety |

flow of gas. Often the patient demonstrates a crowing-like noise called *stridor,* intercostal retractions, and use of the accessory muscles of inspiration. Expiratory dyspnea occurs primarily when there is obstruction to airflow in the lower airways, as in asthma and emphysema, and is characterized by a prolonged expiratory phase.

### Characterizing Dyspnea

When evaluating a patient, whether or not dyspnea is present can be determined by asking, "Do you have any trouble with your breathing?". If the presence of dyspnea is confirmed, it is important to determine the duration and frequency. Is the patient's shortness of breath related to posture, emotion, or abdominal distention? Does it occur at a particular time of the day or night? Determining the severity of the dyspnea is equally important. If the patient responds in the affirmative to the question, "Are you troubled by shortness of breath when hurrying on level ground or walking up a slight hill?", ask the patient, "Do you have to walk slower than people of your age on level ground because of your breathlessness?". Other questions designed to determine the severity of dyspnea include, "Do you ever have to stop and catch your breath after walking a few minutes on level ground?" and "Do you become short of breath while dressing or undressing?".

A type of dyspnea which is characteristic of patients with congestive heart failure or mitral stenosis is *orthopnea.* This is the term used to describe dyspnea which occurs when the individual is at rest in the recumbent position but not when the individual is in the upright position. This experience of dyspnea in the supine position is thought to result from the fact that in the supine position more of the lung is below the level of the heart; hence the higher vascular pressures caused by the cardiac condition are distributed throughout a greater portion of the lung (Lukas, 1970). When the patient is in an upright position, hydrostatic effects lower the pulmonary venous and capillary pressures.

In the normal individual, the vital capacity decreases 5 to 10% when the supine position is assumed. In the individual with congestive heart failure, however, the reduction in vital capacity may be as high as 30% (Hopkins, 1966). In contrast, patients with pulmonary emphysema experience no dyspnea while in the recumbent position. The reason for this is believed to be that the supine position provides better ventilation/perfusion relationships in patients with severely diseased lower lobes (Kory, 1974).

Since orthopnea is relieved by maintaining a semi-vertical position, patients often sleep with multiple pillows under the head and back. A method of determining the severity of the orthopnea is to ask the patient how many pillows are used for sleeping. The condition is then referred to as "two-pillow" or "three-pillow" orthopnea and should be recorded in the patient's record as such.

Another type of dyspnea which commonly occurs in patients with any condition that stresses the left ventrical (pulmonary vascular congestion, congestive heart failure, mitral valve disease) is *paroxysmal nocturnal dyspnea.* In the classic appearance, the patient is suddenly awakened at night by breathlessness so severe that he is forced to sit on the edge of the bed or go open a window in order to relieve the suffocating feeling. Often, both inspiratory and expiratory wheezes can be heard, and the chest is fixed in the inspiratory position. The dyspnea is usually relieved in a few minutes and the patient is able to return to bed.

The mechanism that produces these attacks includes those factors causing orthopnea as well as the hypervolemia resulting from the redistribution of peripheral edema fluid which occurs when the body position is changed from vertical to horizontal (Perera, 1943). The stimulus that actually initiates the attack may be a cough, a startling noise, or anything that increases the heart rate and elevates the pulmonary capillary pressures. Usually, the attack is terminated when the patient sits up and takes a few deep breaths of air.

### Chronic Obstructive Pulmonary Disease

When interviewing the patient, it is important to determine whether the description is one of true paroxysmal nocturnal dyspnea or one of dyspnea associated with chronic obstructive pulmonary disease. The classic appearance of paroxysmal nocturnal dyspnea has been described above; dyspnea secondary to COPD resembles paroxysmal nocturnal dyspnea but is usually associated with cough and sputum production. The patient may get out of bed, but this is to cough up and expectorate the secretions responsible for the dyspnea. Careful questioning can distinguish the cause of the dyspnea. "Do you ever awaken at night and feel as though you need to open a window?" "Does getting up relieve the shortness of breath?" "Do you cough up phlegm on these occasions?" If the patient answers "yes" to this last question, ask, "Does coughing up the phlegm enable you to breath more easily and go back to sleep?".

## Chest Pain

Chest pain is a frequent and more enigmatic symptom which confronts the clinician. Unless caused by obvious trauma, the degree of chest pain is likely to be exaggerated by the patient's fear that it might be the result of heart disease. Because chest pain is often accompanied by no other physical signs, a careful and systematic approach is required to determine its nature and cause. The etiology of chest pain can be divided into five categories: 1) precordial, 2) tracheobronchial, 3) pleuritic, 4) substernal, and 5) musculoskeletal.

### Precordial Pain

Precordial pain is probably the most common type of chest pain of which patients complain. It can be either mild or moderate, and generally it is a short-lasting, sticking or stabbing pain independent of physical activity. It is usually located to the left of the sternum around the area of the cardiac apex. Precordial pain may radiate to other areas of the chest, although it is usually localized. It is seldom the result of any organic heart disease except in acute pericarditis, in which the pain may be severe.

There is a very common type of precordial chest pain which prompts the patient to seek medical attention out of fear of heart disease. In the "precordial catch" or chest wall twinge syndrome (Stegman, 1970), the patient experiences brief periods of sharp pains or "catches" in the anterior chest, usually on the left side. This pain has no association with exercise, although many patients notice this pain when they are hunched over. The pain can last anywhere from fifteen seconds to several minutes and is often aggravated by deep respirations. The exact cause of this pain is unknown, but it is theorized that this kind of chest pain may be the result of costochondral pain or intercostal muscle spasm. Although the condition is harmless, the clinician should reassure the patient that it is not due to heart trouble.

## Tracheobronchial Pain

Tracheobronchial pain is characteristically a burning, substernal pain often exaggerated by deep breathing and coughing. This type of chest pain is most frequently caused by acute tracheitis (inflammation of the trachea); however, the same pain can result from inhalation of noxious fumes, the aspiration of a sharp object, or carcinoma in the trachea or main bronchi. Tracheitis is the result of an upper respiratory infection progressing down into the trachea and large bronchi. Questioning the patient suffering from tracheobronchial chest pain will usually reveal a history of concomitant upper respiratory infection.

## Pleuritic Pain

Pleuritic chest pain is an acute, sharp, and localized pain often precipitated by breathing and motion of the chest. This kind of chest pain results from stimulation of the parietal pleura which, in contrast to the visceral pleura, has sensory innervation and pain endings. Usually the pain is localized to the area overlying the point of pleural involvement, which is usually the bases as most of the respiratory motion occurs here. The pain resulting from diaphragmatic pleurisy or any other disease involving the parietal pleura, however, can be referred to other areas. When the outer 5 to 8 centimeters of the diaphragmatic pleura is stimulated, the pain is located in the lower thoracic and upper abdominal areas. This is due to the fact that the nerves which innervate the peripheral portion of the diaphragmatic pleura, the fifth and sixth intercostal nerves, also innervate the area near the costal margins. Likewise, stimulation of the central part of the diaphragmatic pleura produces pain felt in the neck and shoulder areas because the central portion of the diaphragmatic pleura is innervated by the same nerve which supplies the superior border of the trapezius muscle, and the phrenic nerve. This pattern of referred pleuritic pain is illustrated in *Figure 3-2*. Thus a pain in the neck may be the result of irritation of the diaphragmatic pleura by a lower lobe pneumonia or a subphrenic abscess. Even in severe parenchymal disease, there will not be pleuritic pain unless the process involves the parietal pleura.

The most common causes of pleuritic chest pain are pneumonias caused by gram positive cocci and Klebsiella; gram negative pneumonias are rarely associated with pleuritic pain. Another important cause of pleuritic chest pain is pulmonary embolism. The clinician should suspect a pulmonary embolism in a patient suffering from sharp chest pain who has a history of peripheral vascular disease, has been inactive for a long period of time, and has recently undergone surgery. A young adult presenting with sharp unilateral chest pain in association with dyspnea should suggest a spontaneous pneumothorax. The diagnosis can be confirmed by physical examination and a chest radiograph.

### Substernal Pain

Substernal pain is a significant type of chest pain and is usually caused by cardiovascular conditions such as angina pectoris and myocardial infarction. As the name implies, this pain originates substernally or on the left side of the chest. Substernal chest pain can vary from mild to severe, short-lasting to persistent, and can radiate to the neck, jaws, shoulders, down either arm, or across the anterior chest. The patient often describes the sensation as a tightness, a squeezing, or a heavy feeling in the chest. "It feels like someone is standing on my chest." is the characteristic description of angina pectoris. It is important to remember that

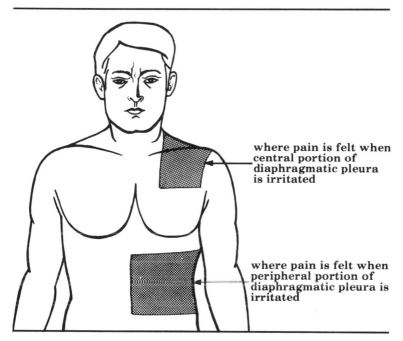

where pain is felt when central portion of diaphragmatic pleura is irritated

where pain is felt when peripheral portion of diaphragmatic pleura is irritated

*Figure 3-2.* Referral of the pain resulting from diseases involving the diaphragmatic pleura. When the central portion of the diaphragmatic pleura is irritated, the pain is referred to the neck and shoulder areas because the central portion of the diaphragmatic pleura and the superior border of the trapezius muscle are both innervated by the phrenic nerve. Stimulation of the peripheral portion of the diaphragmatic pleura results in pain in the lower thoracic and upper abdominal areas because these areas are all innervated by the same nerves, the fifth and sixth intercostal nerves.

the patient often misconstrues this pain as indigestion and denies that a problem exists.

Anginal pain usually originates substernally but can be located anywhere in the chest. Radiation to the neck and/or arms is suggestive of myocardial ischemia. Often the patient has difficulty specifically locating the pain and uses the entire hand to express the area of involvement. In many cases the pain is brought on by exertion or emotion and relieved by rest or nitroglycerin. If the pain lasts longer than one hour, increases in intensity, and is not relieved by nitroglycerin, an acute myocardial infarction should be suspected.

Another cause of substernal pain that is cardiovascular in origin is massive pulmonary embolism, which should be considered when the patient complains of unexplained dyspnea and hemoptysis. The chest pain associated with this condition is often aggravated by inspiration and is sometimes difficult to distinguish from the pain of acute myocardial infarction.

### Musculoskeletal Pain

A type of chest pain that often mimics other types of chest pain is that which is musculoskeletal in etiology. Unfortunately, musculoskeletal pain is often misdiagnosed as pleuritic pain or angina pectoris. In such a case the treatment proves ineffective and the patient may worry needlessly about future "heart attacks."

Rib fracture is a common cause of skeletal pain and should be suspected especially when the patient gives a history of chest trauma. And though patients rarely associate a rib fracture with coughing, repeated severe coughing can fatigue a rib enough to break it, and this should be considered a possible cause of the chest pain. This cause of rib fracture should be especially considered in a case in which there has been no external chest trauma. A summary of the different types of chest pain is found in Table 3-4.

## Characterizing Chest Pain

When interviewing the patient complaining of chest pain, it is important for the clinician to clarify the symptoms so that no important etiology will be overlooked. This clarification can be accomplished by determining certain characteristics of the chest pain:

**Location.** First, the examiner should determine the exact location of the chest pain. A patient's complaint of "pain in my chest" should not suffice. Besides the origin of the pain, the existence and precise location of any radiation of the pain should also be established.

**Severity.** As a means of determining the severity of the chest pain, the interviewer should prompt the patient to describe a typical attack. Noting the patient's facial expressions during his description of a typical attack is one way of evaluating the severity of the pain. Does the patient appear

**Table 3-4. Types of chest pain.**

| Type | Character | Associated conditions |
|------|-----------|----------------------|
| precordial | sticking or stabbing | seldom organic except in acute pericarditis |
| tracheo-bronchial | substernal burning | acute tracheitis, foreign body aspiration, carcinoma |
| pleuritic | sharp, localized, associated with chest movement | gram positive pneumonias, *Klebsiella* pneumonia, pulmonary infarction, pneumothorax |
| substernal | tightness, heavy sensation; can radiate | angina pectoris, myocardial infarction, massive pulmonary embolism |
| musculo-skeletal | sharp, localized (often misinterpreted as pleuritic pain) | rib fracture, chest trauma |

as though he really suffers during an attack, or does he describe a typical attack with an air of nonchalance? How many times has the patient experienced this pain? The duration of the pain should also be ascertained. Is the pain fleeting, persistent, or does it differ from one episode to the next? The duration of the pain should be recorded as specifically as possible in seconds, minutes, hours, etc.

**Character.** The character of the chest pain is the felt quality of the pain (sharp, dull, heavy, crampy, tingling, etc.) as described by the patient. A patient who does not perceive a tightness or burning sensation as pain may respond negatively to the question, "Do you have chest pain?". For this reason a better question might be, "Do you experience any discomfort in your chest?". If so, have the patient describe the discomfort.

**Setting.** The circumstances in which the chest pain occurs should be determined. Does the pain occur during the day, at night, or both? Is the pain related to the patient's posture? Is it noticed during or immediately after physical exertion? Perhaps the pain occurs more often at work under stressful circumstances than at home in a relaxed atmosphere. In order to help distinguish chest pain from indigestion, determine whether the pain is associated with eating. Careful questioning is required to elucidate the essential conditions of the pain when the patient relates that his chest pain is associated with a combination of circumstances.

Determining whether there are any other symptoms associated with the chief complaint of chest pain and what these are can help the clinician determine the cause of the pain. Since many conditions have characteristic symptoms, the patient should be encouraged to describe any other symptoms which occur before, during, or after a typical attack of the chest pain. For example, a history of sharp, localized pleuritic pain which is aggravated by respiration or cough and recent weight loss is suggestive of bronchogenic carcinoma.

**Relieving and Aggravating Factors.** Just as the precipitating factors can point to the cause of chest pain, factors that improve or worsen the pain are also informative. Ask the patient what he does to relieve the pain and what activities or circumstances aggravate the pain. Perhaps the patient is more aware of the pain when walking around or after taking a certain medication. The patient is usually familiar with what relieves the pain.

To summarize, it is important to characterize a symptom of chest pain clearly and completely so that a differential diagnosis can be made. Once the patient has described the pain, specific questions can be asked to explore potential etiologies; eventually enough information will be gathered to suggest a diagnosis.

### Palpitation

"Palpitation," an uncomfortable awareness of the heart beat often described as a pounding, racing, or skipping sensation, is a common complaint. The exact cause of palpitation is unknown. More often than not, it is a result of minor irregularities in cardiac rhythm such as premature beats or paroxysmal tachycardia. The perception of palpitations is thought to be related to the position of the heart inside the chest. When the patient is in a position where the heart is closer to the chest wall, such as the left lateral position, the palpitations may be more easily felt. Some patients are very sensitive to changes in their heart rhythm, while others are totally unaware of any changes. Sometimes an otherwise healthy individual may experience palpitations during times of emotional arousal or anxiety. This sensation is also associated with the ingestion of alcohol, coffee, diet pills, and other stimulatory drugs.

When interviewing the patient complaining of palpitation, determine the duration of each episode and how often the episodes occur. Ask the patient whether the palpitations are noticed with excitement, smoking, coffee, or alcohol. Also have the patient describe the rhythm of the sensation. Does it alternate fast and slow? Perhaps the patient can tap out the rhythm felt. Often an electrocardiogram can identify the precipitating cause.

## Wheezing

Wheezing is an abnormal, musical sound heard during breathing. There have been many theories proposed concerning the origin of wheezes. Historically, wheezes were thought to be generated in much the same way a pipe organ produces sounds. The pitch of the wheeze was believed to be determined by the length and caliber of the airway from which the sound came. Lower-pitched sounds were believed to originate from larger bronchi and higher sounds were thought to come from the smaller peripheral airways. However, several observations contradict this theory on the origin of wheezes. First, the source of a wheeze can be identified with bronchoscopy, and it has been observed that the length of the airway producing the sound has no relation to the pitch of the wheeze. Second, the longest straight pathway in the tracheobronchial tree is less than one foot long, and the pitch of some wheezes is so low that an instrument several feet long would be necessary to reproduce them. Also, the pitch of a wind instrument or pipe will rise when blown with a helium/air mixture, whereas the pitch of a wheeze remains constant when the inspired gas contains helium (Forgacs, 1967).

The mechanics of a wheeze are closer to those of the mouthpiece of an oboe or toy trumpet. This model represents the bronchus as narrowed to the point of closure, with its opposing walls vibrating between the closed and barely open positions during a wheeze (Forgacs, 1978). The pitch of

a wheeze is therefore determined by the mechanical proper-
ties of the structures involved and is independent of the
length of the airway. The velocity of the air is also an important factor in determining the pitch of the wheeze; no musical sound is produced until the linear velocity of the air
through the stenosis reaches a minimum level.

### Expiratory Wheezes

The most common abnormal lung sound is the expiratory
wheeze of diffuse air-flow obstruction. This sound is produced by air being forced under high pressure through airways that are compressed due to a large transmural pressure
gradient. The wheeze of a healthy person performing a
forced expiratory maneuver is similar but higher in pitch
because of a higher linear velocity of air flow. High-pitched
wheezes are common in expiratory flow obstruction such as
that which occurs during an asthma attack. The wheezing in
asthma is not due to peripheral bronchial spasm as once
thought but more often is a sign of fast air flow through
tightly compressed airways (Forgacs, 1978).

Occasionally an expiratory wheeze continues uninter-
rupted into inspiration. This is not actually an inspiratory
wheeze but is a clinical sign of the fact that ventilation of one
part of the lung is out of phase with ventilation of the other
parts of the lung.

Very few patients actually present with a chief complaint
of wheezing. Usually the patient complains of difficulty in
breathing or shortness of breath. And since many patients
diagnose themselves as having asthma, it is important to
take a history of "asthma" loosely. Adult-onset wheezing of
a few months should alert one to the possibility of a mechanical obstruction of the upper airway, trachea, or main-stem
bronchi by a tumor. A long history of wheezing in a patient
with cardiac disease, wheezing which is aggravated when
the patient assumes the supine position, may be indicative of
left ventricular failure. A history of wheezing, chronic sputum production, and dyspnea on exertion in a smoker is
suggestive of emphysema and chronic bronchitis.

### Evaluating Wheezing

In order to determine the etiology of wheezing it is important to ascertain the characteristics of the wheezing. When

interviewing the patient, after the presence of wheezing has been established, determine when the wheezing is the worst. "When do you notice wheezing — during the day or at night?" "Does your chest ever sound wheezy apart from colds?" Some patients confuse wheezing with snoring or bubbling sounds. The examiner might ask, "Does your husband (or wife) regularly complain of your wheezing (not snoring) at night?". If the answer to any of these types of questions is "yes", determine the number of years the condition has been present. Also, ask whether the patient has had an attack of wheezing that led to a feeling of shortness of breath. This is important because wheezing associated with shortness of breath suggests a potential loss of functional capacity. Once the characteristics and the severity of the wheezing have been determined, ask the patient whether these attacks ever required treatment. If so, find out the dosage and frequency of any medication(s) the patient has taken. If the patient has a confirmed history of asthma, a more detailed work-up, including investigation into precipitating factors such as pollen, weather, exercise, aspirin, or animals, should be performed.

It is important when evaluating a patient's wheezing to make a mental note of the characteristics of the breath sounds during auscultation. Determination of the relative pitch and timing of the wheeze (whether it occurs during inspiration, expiration, or both) can help rule out certain disorders.

# Approach to the Physical Examination

*Chapter Four*

## APPROACH TO THE PHYSICAL EXAMINATION

In order to excel as a clinician, one should have a high level of competence in the art of physical examination. In most cases, the physical exam *alone* will not provide the definitive diagnosis; however, in many diseases an evaluation of the physical signs can *lead* to a diagnosis.

The skills utilized in performing the physical exam are different from but just as important as the skills of history-taking. The clinician must use all five senses, sight, touch, hearing, taste, and smell, when physically examining a patient. People vary in their development of these capacities; some are visually perceptive, whereas others are more sensitive to characteristics of sound such as pitch. If one does not feel adept in any one of these areas, improvement can be achieved with practice. Areas of weakness should be identified early so that more time can be devoted to improving them. As development of these skills is usually not part of one's clinical training, many students end up not attaching much importance to the physical examination and as a result fail to gain much from performing them

## Examination Procedure

When learning the skills of physical assessment, it is important to go through the steps of inspection, palpation, percussion, and auscultation in a routine manner. Following the same sequence of evaluation upon entering the room will establish a routine which, once the normal findings have been appreciated, will make it harder to overlook a pathological sign or symptom. There are, however, certain conditions which might necessitate a change in the usual examination procedure. For example, the patient with orthopnea may not tolerate being examined in any position other than sitting up. Other patients may be too ill to be moved at all.

Regardless of the patient's condition, one should be so familiar with the examination procedure that following it correctly and effectively is second nature. Once one has progressed to this point, even the most awkward patient situations will be managed without difficulty.

It is important to keep in mind that people, especially sick people, respond differently to certain situations. Children, as well as the elderly, may act unpredictably in stressful situations such as hospitalization. As the patient is probably apprehensive, emotionally and physically stressed coming into the interview, the examiner should try to make the examination as easy as possible for the patient.

## Examination Room Environment

The room chosen for the examination should be comfortable, warm and well-lighted. If the room is too cool, the patient will shiver, and this will make auscultation of the chest quite difficult. Conversely, if the patient is too warm, normal perspiration might be misconstrued as a pathological sign. Optimally, the examining table should allow the examiner access to both sides of the patient, especially the right side (traditionally, the examiner is on the patient's right during the examination). There may be times when improvisation is required; for example, the examination may have to take place in a bed in the intensive care unit.

Privacy is a must. The patient is more likely to relax if observers are not present. If the patient is a young child, however, a parent may be able to help the child accept and cooperate with the clinician and thereby facilitate the examination. The patient should be completely disrobed and covered with a bed sheet or hospital gown; this provides easy access to the area being examined while covering the rest of the patient's body. For example, when examining the chest, the top part of the gown can be lowered for a few minutes to expose the area of interest without exposing the rest of the body. Erroneous findings may result if the area under examination is not properly exposed.

Adequate exposure of the area being examined should be balanced with respect for the patient's modesty. This is part of maintaining a professional attitude and holds true for both males and females. The clinician's attitude and sense of purpose can be easily detected by the patient; if the patient even suspects an immature attitude, the patient will lose all the confidence (s)he might have had in the examiner.

The patient should *always* be handled with care and respect for the patient's dignity. Touching the patient carefully as one describes a procedure minimizes patient discomfort and enhances the examiner's rapport with the patient. By gently touching the patient on the shoulder or arm, the examiner non-verbally communicates relaxation to the patient which helps abolish some of the patient's anxieties.

By the time the physical examination is to be performed, a carefully taken history should have divulged any particular areas of tenderness the patient might have. At times, palpation of tender areas may be unavoidable. In these instances, it is important to warn the patient that the necessary procedure might hurt. This simple but effective technique also helps the patient gain more confidence in the examiner. In fact, the patient should be informed about what is going to be involved prior to any procedure because no one, especially a sick patient, likes surprises.

One's attitude during the exam should be professional and objective, but not always serious. A friendly smile or light comment will go far towards making the patient feel that the examiner is a real person and relieving any tension that the patient might have.

## Measuring Vital Signs

Measurement of the patient's vital signs should be a routine part of every physical examination. These include temperature, pulse, respirations, and blood pressure. Often these values can be found in the patient's chart; if not, these parameters should be measured at the beginning of the examination.

The following section discusses the rationale for obtaining each of the vital signs, the proper procedures, and the clinical significance of abnormal values.

## Temperature

Since the measurement of body temperature is a useful aid in the evaluation of disease and has been such ever since Galileo invented the thermometer, the patient's temperature should be recorded in the patient's medical record.

Normally, body temperature is maintained relatively constant by a part of the brain called the hypothalamus, which regulates heat loss and production. The hypothalamus and the rest of the nervous system keep body temperature stable by varying the degree of peripheral vasoconstriction or vasodilation, thereby influencing the amount of heat lost from the surface of the body. There are a number of physiologic conditions which can increase body temperature, including food digestion, exercise, ovulation, and pregnancy. Knowledge of the presence of these possible causes of fever can help the clinician evaluate the complaint of "fever" in the patient.

There are three methods used to clinically assess the patient's body temperature — oral, rectal, and axillary. The oral method is used most frequently. In this method, the bulb of the thermometer is placed under the tongue for at least three minutes and then the thermometer is read. The mean normal oral temperature is 98.6°F. or 37°C. Since one should allow for some fluctuation, the normal range of oral temperature should be considered to extend from 97°F. to 100°F. The oral thermometer reading may be inaccurate if the patient has not kept the mouth closed for the prescribed length of time. Also, if the patient recently ingested a hot or cold substance, this will affect the temperature. This method of determining body temperature is unsafe to use with uncooperative patients or with very young children who may bite and break the thermometer.

Body temperature obtained rectally is usually slightly higher (about 0.7°F.) than the oral temperature. However, there are some individuals whose oral temperature is higher than their rectal temperature. The rectal temperature is less variable than the oral temperature and is considered to be more reflective of the "core" temperature. The rectal method of measuring body temperature is preferred with children or those patients who cannot keep the mouth closed during the measurement.

The third clinically used method for taking the patient's body temperature is the axillary method. This method involves placing the the bulb of the thermometer high in the axilla and holding the arm against the chest for a minimum of five minutes. The axillary method is considered by many clinicians to be the least accurate because tissues at a distance from the body core are cooler. The average axillary temperature is about 1°F. lower than the oral temperature. The three methods of measuring body temperature are summarized in Table 4-1.

**Table 4-1. Methods of measuring body temperature and associated normal temperature range and accuracies.**

| Method | Normal range of temperature | Accuracy |
|---|---|---|
| oral | 97.0 — 100°F<br>36.1 — 37.7°C | ++ |
| rectal | 97.7 — 100.7°F<br>36.5 — 38.2°C | +++ |
| axillary | 96.0 — 99.0°F<br>35.5 — 37.2°C | + |

Regardless of the method used for determining the patient's temperature, there is no one "normal" body temperature. In fact, there is a daily rhythmic change in body temperature of 2 to 3°F. For a person who is awake during the day and sleeps at night, the highest temperature is usually between 8 and 11 PM, and the lowest is during sleep between 4 and 6 AM. The usual explanation for this is that the higher temperatures are the result of food digestion and muscle activity, and the lowest temperature occurs when the body's metabolic rate is at a minimum. Also, some healthy individuals have a temperature consistently below normal, and if the environment is warm, the patient's temperature may be as high as 99.6°F. An accurate oral temperature consistently below 97°F. or higher than 100°F. should be considered abnormal.

The temperature record in the patient's chart can provide valuable information regarding the illness of the patient. Abnormally high body temperature can be caused by either increased heat production or impairment of heat elimination. There are a myriad of conditions which can result in fever, and it is not within the scope of this text to include a discussion of these specific causes. Suffice it to say that the temperature is seldom diagnostic in and of itself. However, the type of fever can be characteristic of the general cause of the fever (infection, CNS disorders, or blood diseases). One type of fever is the *continuous fever (Figure 4-1)*, in which the temperature remains consistently elevated during any 24-hour period. Although it can fluctuate over several hours, continuous fever is probably the most common type; it is seen in minor infections and some cases of head injury. In *intermittent fever (Figure 4-2)*, the temperature is elevated at some time during each day but can fall to normal or subnormal levels during the same 24-hour period. This type of fever commonly occurs with infection. *Remittant fever (Figure 4-3)* is characterized by marked fluctuations in temperature each day, with no normal readings. This pattern is seen in typhoid fever and differs from that in continuous fever, in which variations in temperature are slight. *Relapsing fever (Figure 4-4)* is characterized by short febrile periods interspersed with periods of normal temperature lasting one or more days. This type of fever is seen in Hodgkin's disease.

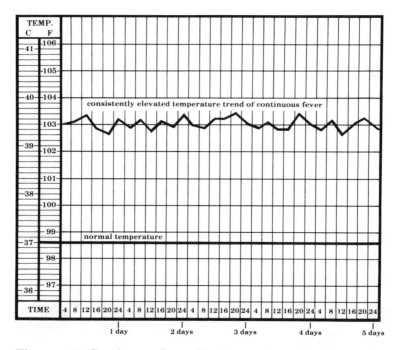

***Figure 4-1.*** Continuous fever. The temperature remains consistently elevated during any 24-hour period with slight fluctuations.

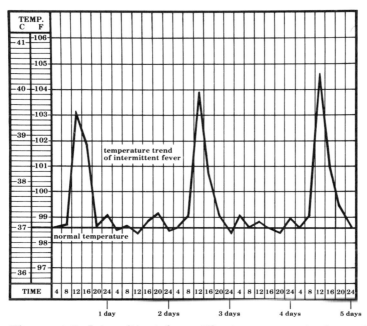

***Figure 4-2.*** Intermittent fever. The temperature is elevated at some time each day but falls to normal or subnormal levels within the same 24-hour period.

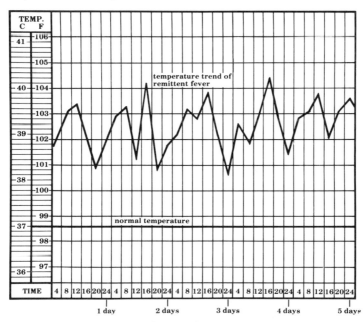

***Figure 4-3.*** Remittent fever. Characterized by marked fluctuations each day with no normal readings.

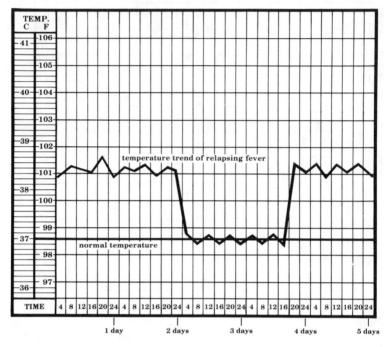

***Figure 4-4.*** Relapsing fever. Characterized by short febrile periods interspersed with periods of one or more days of normal temperature.

## Pulse

Palpation of the pulse should also be a part of the physical examination, and special attention should be paid to the rate, rhythm, and character of the pulse. Customarily, the radial artery over the wrist is used to palpate the pulse, although any artery can be used if necessary. When determining the pulse rate, count the pulse for one full minute using the fingertips and not the thumb (the thumb has a palpable pulse of its own).

### Rate

In adults at rest, the normal rate ranges from 60 to 100 beats per minute; however, the pulse rate varies with age, sex, emotional status, and physical activity. In well-conditioned athletes, a rate as low as 50 beats per minute is not unusual. In infants and children the rate is higher, varying from 90 to 120 beats per minute with rates of 130 to 140 beats per minute not considered abnormal.

When the heart rate is faster than normal, *tachycardia* is said to be present. There are many causes of tachycardia, including the medical interview itself. If the pulse rate is high initially, recheck it at the end of the examination. Persistent tachycardia is found in severe anemias, massive hemorrhage, hyperthyroidism, certain types of cardiac arrhythmias, and high fever. In most febrile conditions the pulse rate increases five to ten beats per minute for each °F above normal.

An abnormally slow heart rate is called *bradycardia.* This can occur in patients with increased intracranial pressure, obstructive jaundice, and some arrhythmias such as complete heart block. In most cases, no treatment is required for bradycardia. When treatment is warranted, treating the underlying cause of the bradycardia is indicated.

### Rhythm

If the rhythm of the heart and pulse is regular, the patient has a *normal sinus rhythm.* If there is an irregularity, a *dysrhythmia* is present. The more common rhythm disturbances can be detected by palpating the pulse. It should be mentioned that auscultation of the heart and an electrocardiogram (ECG) are more accurate methods of evaluating the rhythm.

### Character

The character of the pulse is dependent on the magnitude of the pulse pressure (the difference between the systolic and diastolic blood pressures) and the rate at which this difference increases and decreases. The character of the pulse can range from feeble and thready to forceful and bounding.

### Abnormalities of the Pulse

There are several abnormalities of the pulse beat which warrant the clinician's attention. *Pulsus parvus* is a small, weak pulse that seems to rise and fall slowly in magnitude. It occurs when the pulse pressure is narrow due to an increased peripheral vascular resistance or a low left ventricular stroke volume as in aortic stenosis.

Paradoxical pulse *(pulsus paradoxus)* is characterized by a decrease in the force (not the rate) of the pulse almost to the point of disappearance during the inspiratory phase of respiration; the pulse beat can be felt to regain force during expiration. This will occur in normal individuals during a sustained, deep inspiration. However, pulsus paradoxus occurring during quiet respiration is abnormal. This phenomenon is the result of an increase in the intrathoracic pressure causing a pooling of blood in the expanded lungs which results in a decreased venous return to the heart, a decrease in cardiac output, and lower blood pressure. A paradoxical pulse is best confirmed with a sphygmomanometer. The blood pressure cuff is placed around the arm and the peak systolic pressure is measured during inspiration. A pressure drop of 5 mm Hg during inspiration is considered normal, but if the systolic pressure falls more than 10 mm Hg during inspiration, the pulse is paradoxical. Pulsus paradoxus is found in patients with constrictive pericarditis, pericardial effusion, heart failure, severe emphysema, and asthma.

Another pulse abnormality is *pulsus alternans,* which is characterized by strong beats alternating with weak beats. This phenomenon, too, is best detected with a sphygmomanometer. Initially, only the stronger beats are heard. Then, as the pressure in the cuff is lowered, weaker beats will be heard between the stronger beats and the rate will appear to double. Pulsus alternans is observed in severe hypertension, left ventricular failure, and coronary artery disease.

## Blood Pressure

The final component of the patient's vital signs to be measured is the arterial blood pressure. The patient should be relaxed and comfortable when his blood pressure is being measured as blood pressure can be elevated by anxiety. The patient should be either seated or in the recumbent position and the arm should be slightly flexed, supported on a firm surface, and free of clothing.

It is advisable to take the blood pressure twice during the examination, once at the beginning and then again later in the exam, because the initial measurement may be falsely elevated or depressed by a number of different factors including: tension, anxiety, anger, physical exertion, pain, smoking, or being too hot or too cold. After the patient has had a chance to relax, repeating the measurement should provide a more reliable result.

Blood pressure may be measured with either of two types of sphygmomanometer, the aneroid type or the mercury type. The aneroid manometer has a flexible, spring-supported top that responds to changes in pressure. Mercury is used in the other type of manometer because the density of mercury is such that at ordinary pressures it assumes a height that is easily read. It makes no difference which instrument is used as long as the instrument used is accurately calibrated and properly used.

### Procedure

Measuring blood pressure is quite simple. Begin by deflating the pressure cuff completely before wrapping it snugly around the arm. The lower edge of the cuff should be 2 to 3 centimeters above the antecubital fossa with the rubber tubing along the medial aspect of the arm. Palpate the radial pulse, close the valve on the bulb, and rapidly inflate the cuff to a pressure about 25 mm Hg above the point at which the radial pulse disappears. As the cuff is deflated slowly, the pressure at which the pulse reappears is the *palpatory systolic pressure.*

The *auscultory method* is then used to determine both the systolic and diastolic pressures. In this method, the bell or diaphragm of the stethoscope is placed over the brachial artery, which is just medial to the biceps tendon. The bell or diaphragm should not be touching the cuff or the tubes in order to avoid any artifactual noise. The valve is then closed and the cuff is inflated to a pressure about 30 mm Hg over the palpatory systolic pressure. As the pressure is released slowly, the pressure at which the first sound is heard through the stethoscope is the *systolic pressure.* As the cuff is deflated, the sounds will become damped and dull and then disappear. The pressure at which the sound completely disappears is the *diastolic pressure.* The patient's blood pressure is then recorded as a fraction, with the systolic pressure over the diastolic pressure — 120/80, for example.

### Auscultory Gap

In some patients a phenomenon known as *auscultory gap* occurs. The clinician first detects the pulse sounds at a high pressure level, then the sounds disappear only to return at a lower pressure level. For example, the sounds may first be heard at 170 mm Hg. These sounds persist until the pressure falls to 160 mm Hg, at which time the sounds disappear. They reappear at 130 mm Hg and continue until the diastolic pressure is reached. In this case the auscultory gap is the difference in pressure between 160 mm Hg and 130 mm Hg. If in this case the cuff were only inflated to 150 mm Hg, the examiner might be misled to thinking that 130 mm Hg is the systolic pressure rather than 170 mm Hg.

Determination of blood pressure in the legs is not routinely performed. However, comparing the blood pressure in the leg to the blood pressure in the arm can help to determine whether arterial occlusion is present; there is a possibility that this condition is present in the patient if the blood pressure is lower in the leg than in the arm. The blood pressure in the leg is determined by applying the cuff around the lower third of the thigh and placing the bell of the stethoscope over the popliteal artery. If a standard size cuff is used, the systolic pressure in the leg may be 20 to 30 mm Hg higher than in the arm. With a wide cuff (20 cm), this discrepancy is less.

### Normal Findings

Normal blood pressure in the adult varies over a wide range. What is normal in terms of blood pressure depends upon sex, race, physical activity, and the degree of tension present. Obese extremities will often cause a falsely elevated systolic pressure; this occurs because the cuff pressure must overcome the resistance of the tissues before compressing the selected artery. The accepted range for normal systolic pressure is 110 to 150 mm Hg; 90 mm Hg is considered the normal upper limit of the diastolic pressure. As a person ages, the blood pressure will rise due to gradual arteriosclerosis. Some patients have a slightly lower blood pressure with the systolic pressure around 90 mm Hg; this poses no serious health threat unless accompanied by other symptoms.

### Pulse Pressure

The *pulse pressure* is the difference between the systolic and diastolic pressures. In an individual with a blood pressure of 120/80 mm Hg, the pulse pressure is 40 mm Hg.

There are two major factors which affect the pulse pressure: 1) the stroke volume output of the heart and 2) the compliance of the arteries. The pulse pressure is directly related to the former and indirectly related to the latter. As the stroke volume output increases, the pulse pressure increases, and in conditions which result in decreased stroke volume output, the pulse pressure decreases accordingly. The compliance of the arteries is significantly affected by the mean arterial pressure (see below) and the distensibility of the arterial walls. As the mean arterial pressure increases, the compliance decreases slightly. Thus the pulse pressure is increased in an individual who has high arterial pressures with a normal stroke volume. As the distensibility of the arterial walls decreases so does the compliance of the arteries. As a person ages, the arterial walls lose much of their elastic tissue, resulting in a decrease in the distensibility of the arterial walls and the compliance of the arterial system. This will cause the pulse pressure to increase.

### *Mean Arterial Pressure*

The mean arterial pressure can be calculated by dividing the pulse pressure by 3 and adding this value to the diastolic pressure. For a blood pressure of 120/80, the mean arterial pressure is:

$$\frac{40}{3} + 80 = 93 \text{ mm Hg.}$$

### *Variations in Blood Pressure*

Changes in blood pressure can occur with a number of cardiac dysrhythmias. In a condition of premature ventricular contractions, for example, the ventricles can become overfilled during the compensatory pause, which is the time delay that often follows a premature contraction; if so, the subsequent beat will result in a systolic pressure higher than that of the other beats. Causes of high blood pressure (hypertension) include: essential hypertension, chronic glomerulonephritis, coarctation of the aorta, and renal artery stenosis. Among the causes of low blood pressure (hypotension) are Addison's disease, acute myocardial infarction, and shock.

### Sources of Error in Blood Pressure Measurement

There are several common sources of error in blood pressure measurement of which the clinician should be aware: 1) the fit of the cuff, 2) the relationship of cuff size to limb size, 3) anxiety, and 4) failure to recognize an auscultory gap.

1. If the blood pressure cuff is wrapped too loosely around the patient's arm, erroneously high values will result.

2. Discrepancies between the cuff size and the limb size can result in inaccurate measurements. As previously mentioned, falsely elevated values are not unusual in the obese arm or thigh, particularly if an undersized cuff is used. If the cuff is too large for the limb, false low values will result.

3. Anxiety in the patient may cause an elevated blood pressure. If the pressure is initially high, recheck the pressure later in the examination.

4. Failure to recognize the presence of an auscultory gap will result in inaccurate systolic pressure readings. False low values will be obtained if in search of the palpatory systolic pressure the pressure in the cuff is increased to a point within the range of the gap but not high enough to determine the true systolic pressure.

# Inspection

*Chapter Five*

**INSPECTION**

Inspection is the collection of information on physical signs from visual observation of the patient. Of the traditional methods of physical examination, inspection is probably the most difficult to learn, but it yields the most information. It is difficult to learn for several reasons. First, the art of observation is not emphasized in school, and as a result, many students do not deem it worthy of much attention. More often than not, clinical instructors attach greater significance to the mechanical skills of percussion and auscultation. Secondly, people have a tendency to see only those things that mean something to them. If the clinician is familiar with the physical signs associated with a particular disease, he will probably be able to recognize them when examining the patient; if (s)he isn't familiar with the signs, (s)he probably won't recognize them. Thus improvement of the clinician's inspection skills can only come with an increase in experience and knowledge of diseases and their symptoms.

The process of inspection actually begins during the taking of the medical history. During this time, one should observe the responsiveness of the patient, the speech pattern, body movements, and some personality traits. Though one might observe the patient more closely later in the exam, staying alert to any conspicuous abnormalities during the taking of the history can also be informative. As the history evolves into more of a conversation, the patient is less likely to be aware of being observed. In many cases, one can accomplish much of the inspection during palpation and auscultation; however, the clinician should be trying during the taking of the history to organize any significant physical findings observed into an educated diagnosis.

Inspection is usually performed with the patient sitting in a comfortable position, although some prefer that the patient be in the supine position. Whichever position is chosen, using the same position as much as possible, will accustom the clinician to viewing the patient from a particular angle and thereby enable him to more readily notice any abnormalities.

One aspect of the inspection skill which the clinician should cultivate is the ability to observe when the patient is least suspicious. If the patient is aware of being observed, then his or her actions and mannerisms may change to conform to what he or she thinks is expected; the patient may no longer respond in a natural, unselfconscious manner. For example, if the patient knows that his respiratory rate is being assessed, it is not likely that the rate will be normal, either because the patient is anxious or because the patient might try to falsify the results in an effort to gain disability benefits.

There is an abundance of information which can be obtained before laying the first hand on the patient. The following things should be observed in order for the examination to be complete: 1) mental status, 2) nutritional status, 3) posture, 4) skin, 5) neck, 6) extremities, 7) thorax and bony structures, and 8) the rate and pattern of breathing.

## Mental Status

Evaluation of the mental status of the patient actually begins during the interview. Simply from talking with the patient one can determine whether the patient is hyperactive, retarded, or withdrawn. From the patient's responses to the questions, one can tell whether the patient is alert or disoriented. Are the patient's responses appropriate to the questions? If the interview was not performed prior to the physical exam and this is the first meeting with the patient, upon entering the room one can at least determine whether the patient is conscious, semi-comatose, or comatose.

The patient's behavior is often a reflection of his mental status. Behavior is a form of nonverbal communication and as such can at times be more informative than what the patient says. Because the manner in which the patient acts can be indicative of the presence of disturbances at many different levels, significant information can be gleaned from close observation of the patient during the interview. For example, emotional or physical problems may be manifested by slowed movements, tremors, or undue tension such as crying. The mannerisms which the patient displays, such as facial expressions, give clues about the patient's personality or feelings at that moment. The patient may greet the staff with a friendly smile or may appear very depressed.

If the examination takes place in an outpatient clinic setting, the patient's appearance can provide information on the patient's self-image. Is the patient neatly dressed? Does he have a scraggly beard? Does it seem as if the patient cares about his or her appearance? The value the patient places on his own appearance is related to his self-esteem.

## Nutritional Status

As part of the general survey, the patient's nutritional status should be assessed. The patient is usually evaluated in general terms such as being underweight or overweight, and this is generally obvious after a few minutes in the patient's room.

There are, of course, different degrees of the condition in both categories. The patient may be mildly underweight, which usually presents no problem, severely underweight (cachectic), or anywhere in between. If the patient is underweight, it should be determined whether he or she has always been slender or if there has been a recent weight loss. An unusual or rapid loss in weight can be attributed to any number of causes, including hyperthyroidism, malignancy, mental depression, or nutritional depletion. Therefore, it is important to view a state of underweight in terms of the patient's average weight. Those people who are naturally underweight are classified as *ectomorphs*. These people are thin with small bone structures. Ectomorphs usually have a thin chest with prominent ribs and a flat abdomen.

The person with an average body build is called a *mesomorph*. This individual typically has larger bones, broad shoulders, a flat abdomen, and greater muscle mass than the ectomorph.

Since obesity has almost reached epidemic proportions in our society, it is not unusual to see the overweight individual as a patient. The overweight person, or *endomorph*, has a large, soft, bulging body. The extremities, as well as the neck, are short and thick, and the face is round. The muscle development may be good, but it is difficult to distinguish muscle mass from fat.

Obesity may be either exogenous or endogenous. The most common cause of exogenous obesity is simply overeating. In these individuals, the fat distribution is generalized over the entire body. Endogenous obesity, on the other hand, may be attributed to certain endocrine disorders such as hyperthy-roidism and Cushing's syndrome. In the person with endo-genous obesity, the fat is localized to certain regions of the body such as the girdle area, while the extremities are more lean.

## Posture

Upon entering the patient's room, the clinician should quickly assess the posture of the patient, for it may be sug-gestive of certain abnormalities. If the patient is leaning forward over the bedside table and mentions that breathing is easier in this position, this may be suggestive of chronic obstructive pulmonary disease or congestive heart failure. If the patient is leaning to one side and cannot sit up straight, there may be some degree of scoliosis present. An inability to turn the head without having to turn the entire upper body because the neck is rigid may be indicative of cervical arthri-tis. Thus, taking note of the posture of the patient at the time of the examination, while not always diagnostic, can be very suggestive of certain disease possibilities.

## Skin

Inspection of the skin is an important part of any physical examination. When the clinician is examining the pulmo-nary patient, inspection of the entire area of the skin is usually not required; a satisfactory examination of the skin can be accomplished while inspecting the anterior and pos-terior chest, neck, and extremities.

Evaluation of the skin consists primarily of inspection, with palpation being used to confirm any significant find-ings. No special instruments are used to evaluate the skin; however, this should not detract from the importance of careful skin examination.

In order to ascertain whether a lesion represents a skin disorder or is simply a normal variation, adequate light is a must. An evenly, preferably natural-lighted room is required for examination. Without good lighting, it is difficult for the examiner to distinguish pallor from cyanosis or petechiae from freckles.

## Color

The first thing the clinician usually notices is the color of the skin. The normal skin pigments are melanin, hemoglobin, and the carotenoids. Most individuals have all of these pigments; however, the amounts of these pigments in the skin vary from person to person. Skin tones can vary from pallor secondary to anemia to erythemia (redness) secondary to fever or sunburn.

Changes in skin color can be the result of there being significant quantities of some pigments not normally found in large amounts in the skin. For example, increased levels of bilirubin will give a yellow tone to the skin which is indicative of jaundice. In dark-skinned persons, this will be more evident in the conjunctivae and the oral mucosa.

## Cyanosis

Not uncommon in patients with pulmonary disease is *cyanosis*, which results in a bluish color of the skin. This is the result of an abnormal level (at least 5 grams/100 ml) of deoxyhemoglobin in the blood. Cyanosis is best evaluated in areas where the coverings over the capillaries in the skin and mucous membranes are the thinnest, such as in the gums, earlobes, and lips. Cyanosis can be either central or peripheral in appearance. Central cyanosis is commonly seen in advanced pulmonary disease, such as emphysema or chronic bronchitis, and congenital heart diseases with right-to-left shunting. Peripheral cyanosis (acrocyanosis) is seen only in the extremities, ears, and lips and is caused by a reduction in the systemic blood flow resulting from a decreased cardiac output.

The severity of cyanosis and the degree to which it can be recognized are related to the hemoglobin concentration. If in the anemic patient, whose hemoglobin concentration might be 8 grams/100 ml (8 gm%) of blood, the hemoglobin were 50% saturated, there would be 4 grams of deoxyhemoglobin. In such a case, cyanosis would not be readily apparent, but the patient would be hypoxic because of the reduced oxygen-carrying capacity. Conversely, if in the patient with polycythemia, whose hemoglobin concentration might be 20 grams/100 ml (20 gm%) of blood, the hemoglobin were 50% saturated, there would be 10 grams of deoxyhemoglobin. In this case, the patient would develop cyanosis more quickly but might not be hypoxic. It is important to remember that tissue hypoxia does not necessarily result in cyanosis, and the mere presence of cyanosis does not indicate the presence of hypoxia.

During the examination of the skin, the presence of any scars resulting from either surgery or injury, particularly on the neck or thorax, should be noted. Any previous surgical procedures should have already been described in the history, so a scar from a thoracotomy, for example, found when inspecting the thorax should not be surprising.

## Neck

One will soon learn that this small area of body tissue contains many important structures, and changes in these structures are often indicative of problems in other areas of the body, especially the chest.

Examination of the neck is accomplished by inspection and palpation, with auscultation being occasionally helpful. Inspection of the neck should be performed with the patient relaxed and in an upright position under good lighting. The procedure is made easier if the patient's head is turned to the side opposite from that being viewed. This helps accentuate muscles, cartilages, and pulsations in the neck.

### Size and Shape

The size and shape of the neck will vary with the body type of the patient. In some cases, this variability can limit the effectiveness of the examination. In the ectomorph, the neck is long and "swan-like," making the anatomical structures within, easily discernable. Severe malnutrition may simulate this appearance also. In contrast, the neck of the endomorph is typically a short, thick "bull neck;" severe emphysema may produce the same appearance. The subcutaneous fat that is present in this type of neck may make it difficult to adequately evaluate the contained structures. The size and shape of the neck should correlate to the stature of the individual; a deviation should raise suspicion of possible disease.

## *Mobility*

Inspection of the neck should also include an evaluation of the neck's mobility. Any abnormal position of the head or neck is readily apparent upon entering the room and should be noted. A limitation of motion, however, can be less obvious to the observer. Evaluating the range of motion of the neck is easily performed by having the patient move the head up and down and from side to side. If there is limited movement and the patient complains of stiffness, arthritis is a possibility. Myasthenia gravis might be suspected if the patient has difficulty holding the head in one position for more than a short time.

## *Symmetry*

One of the major functions of inspection is the detection of abnormalities causing asymmetry between the two sides of the neck. This technique consists of having the patient seated comfortably so that the muscles in both sides of the neck are relaxed. The examiner should be positioned in front of the individual to compare the two sides of the neck.

Asymmetry of the neck is most often due to masses or enlargement of one of the normal structures such as the thyroid gland, lymph nodes, or neck muscles. To detect this, the clinician should inspect the submandibular and suprasternal areas for any swelling. Then the bases of the neck, including the supraclavicular fossae areas, are compared. One should not forget to inspect the back of the neck because disease of the vertebrae can result in asymmetry.

## *Scars*

The presence of and reasons for any scars on the neck should have been mentioned in the history. If a scar was overlooked during the history-taking, then this is an appropriate time to inquire about the past medical history related to the scar. It is not unusual to see a patient with a cicatrix from a tracheotomy or a thyroidectomy. One reason to have the patient extend the head backward for optimal visualization is that a scar from a skillful surgeon might be hidden in one of the creases in the neck and easily overlooked.

### Pulsations

It is important to inspect the neck for any abnormal pulsations of the jugular veins or carotid arteries. The jugular veins should not be obvious upon inspection of the quietly breathing, upright patient. If there is persistent distention of the external jugular veins, it is most likely secondary to right heart failure. Likewise, visible pulsations of the carotid arteries should not be present except in the very thin individual. Carotid artery pulsations can, however, be the result of emotional stress or exercise; but they can also be the result of a more serious condition such as hypertension, anemia, or aortic regurgitation.

### Laryngeal Cartilages

Of the structures comprising the larynx, the largest and most visible cartilage is the thyroid cartilage. Otherwise known as the "Adam's apple," this cartilage is more prominent in males than in females. Normally, it should be midline and move upward like the thyroid gland when the patient swallows. Sometimes the laryngeal cartilages can be rotated, giving a false impression of tracheal deviation.

### Accessory Muscles of Inspiration

While observing the patient breathing quietly, it should be noted whether there is any use of the accessory muscles of inspiration. Use of the accessory muscles indicates the patient is working harder than normal to breathe. The accessory muscles which show respiratory activity the most are the scalenes, the sternocleidomastoids, and the trapezius muscles. A more detailed description of the accessory muscles of inspiration is provided later in this chapter.

## Extremities

There are many disease processes, both cardiac and pulmonary in origin, with manifestations in the extremities. When evaluating the hands and feet, inspection is a very important procedure. During inspection, it is important to compare the extremity with its counterpart on the opposite side of the patient's body in order to determine symmetry and to detect abnormalities that may affect only one side. Examination of the extremities should be systematic, beginning with the fingers and toes and progressing up the arms and legs respectively.

## Nails

The nails and the nail beds of the hands should always be inspected. As previously mentioned, the nail beds are sensitive to the discoloration of anemia, polycythemia, and cyanosis. Discoloration of the nails may be due to occupational exposure to chemicals. Also, a chronic cigarette smoker often has yellow stains on his finger tips.

## Digital Clubbing

Another important clinical sign associated with the fingers and toes is digital clubbing. This sign is characterized by loss of the normal angle at the base of the nails. Normally, the angle between the root of the nail and the nail bed is about 160°. Over a period of months or years, the soft tissue covering the root of the nail bed can hypertrophy and this angle becomes 180° or more (see *Figure 5-1*). As the clubbing progresses, the nail thickens and the distal phalanx enlarges and assumes a bulbous appearance.

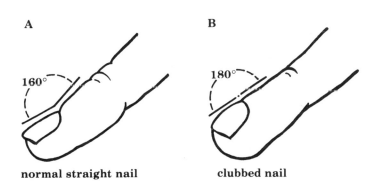

normal straight nail          clubbed nail

*Figure 5-1.* Digital clubbing. (**A**) In the normal finger, the angle formed between the root of the nail and the nail bed is no greater than 160°. (**B**) As clubbing progresses, this angle approaches 180° or more.

The exact mechanism of digital clubbing is presently unknown. But regardless of the underlying cause, all types of clubbing show the same pathological changes. The development of digital clubbing has been thought to be associated with tissue hypoxia and the resultant increase in the number of arteriovenous anastamoses in the limbs. This is shown to be true when right-to-left shunts are experimentally induced in laboratory animals. Tissue hypoxia is a plausible mechanism in pulmonary or cardiovascular conditions; however, this hypothesis does not explain how patients with ulcerative colitis (another kind of condition with which clubbing is associated) develop clubbing.

Another theory of the pathogenesis of digital clubbing is that this condition results from an increase in blood flow to the extremities — more blood flows to the extremities than is necessary to meet the demands of the tissues, with the result that the growth of the digital tissues is increased. Some of the more common causes of digital clubbing are listed in Table 5-1.

**Table 5-1. Causes of digital clubbing.**

| Pulmonary | Cardiovascular |
|---|---|
| bronchiectasis | cyanotic, congenital heart disease |
| emphysema | advanced cor pulmonale |
| bronchogenic carcinoma | subacute bacterial endocarditis |
| pleural mesothelioma | pulmonary arteriovenous fistula |
| **Gastrointestinal** | **Hepatic** |
| regional enteritis | biliary cirrhosis |
| ulcerative colitis | liver abscess |
| dysentery | |
| **Congenital** | |
| pachyderma periostitis | |

### Edema

If edema of the skin (accumulation of fluid in the subcutaneous tissues) is present, it can be easily recognized in the hands and feet. With inspection it is noticed that the edematous area has lost its normal curvature and landmarks; the wrist bones and/or ankle bones will disappear. The skin is often stretched and shiny and in some cases small cracks in the skin may develop, from which fluid oozes.

The causes of peripheral edema formation are too numerous to be covered within the scope of this text. In general, however, edema can be caused by increased venous pressure, as found in right-sided heart failure, decreased lymphatic return secondary to tumors or inflammation, and electrolyte imbalances such as hypoalbuminemia or hypernatremia.

## Thorax

### Reference Lines

Before beginning a discussion on examination of the thorax, it is appropriate to review the anatomy and important landmarks of the chest so that the precise location of a breath sound or lesion can be determined. To help in this process, a number of imaginary lines on the anterior, lateral, and posterior chest wall are used as reference points. The following vertical lines are useful on the anterior chest *(Figure 5-2)*:

**Midsternal line:** The midsternal line is a vertical line through the middle of the sternum.

**Midclavicular lines:** The midclavicular lines run parallel to the midsternal line and extend downward from the midpoint of each clavicle.

On the lateral chest wall, three vertical lines are useful *(Figure 5-3)*:

**Anterior axillary line:** The anterior axillary line is an imaginary line which runs vertically from the anterior axillary fold along the anterolateral chest on both sides of the body.

**Posterior axillary line:** The posterior axillary line runs vertically from the posterior axillary fold along the posterolateral chest on both sides of the body.

**Midaxillary line:** The midaxillary line is an imaginary vertical line extending from the apex of each axilla midway between the anterior and the posterior axillary lines. To locate these three lines, the arm must be raised directly from the lateral chest wall. If the arm is moved either anteriorly or posteriorly, the normal position of the axilla relative to the chest wall will be altered.

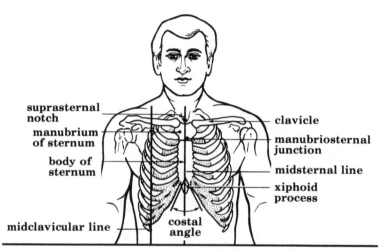

**Figure 5-2.** Bony landmarks and reference lines of the anterior thorax.

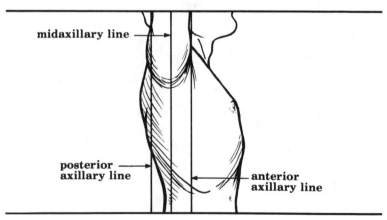

**Figure 5-3.** Reference lines on the lateral chest wall.

There are also three useful imaginary reference lines on the posterior chest wall *(Figure 5-4):*

**Midspinal line:** The midspinal line runs down the posterior spinous processes of the vertebrae, dividing the back into two equal halves.

**Midscapular lines:** Each midscapular line intersects the apex and the inferior angle of the scapula and runs parallel to the midspinal line. The midscapular lines are not used as often as other lines of reference because of the mobility of the scapulae. If these reference lines are used, the patient should be sitting or standing erect with the arms at the sides of the body.

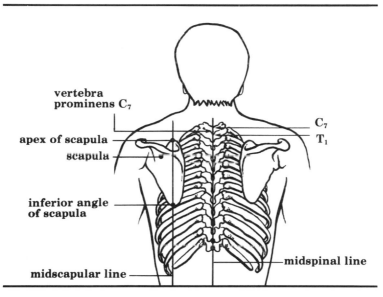

*Figure 5-4.* Bony landmarks and reference lines on the posterior chest wall.

### Bony Landmarks

On the anterior chest there are two important bony landmarks *(Figure 5-2).* The first is the *suprasternal notch,* which marks the top of the manubrium. The other is the *manubriosternal junction* or "angle of Louis," which is the joint between the manubrium and the body of the sternum (gladiolus). The manubriosternal junction lies at the level at which the second ribs attach to the sternum and is visible in most persons. When counting ribs, this landmark is a convenient starting point. The angle of Louis also approximates the level of the bifurcation of the trachea at the *carina*.

To help identify thoracic vertebrae and posterior ribs, the spinous process of the seventh cervical vertebra (vertebra prominens) is a useful landmark *(Figure 5-4)*. This vertebra ($C_7$) can be identified when the patient flexes the neck anteriorly.

These imaginary lines and anatomical landmarks serve as reference points when describing the location of a lesion. An accurate description of the location of a lesion would read something like: "three centimeters medial to the left midclavicular line at the level of the fifth intercostal space". With a description of this kind, any other staff who might need to see or feel the lesion at a later date would be able to identify the exact location.

### Lobar Anatomy

During examination of the respiratory system, the clinician should have a mental image of the surface projections of the lungs and the lobar anatomy within the chest. The apex of each lung extends about 1 1/2 inches above the clavicle. In the anterior chest, the inferior borders of the lungs cross the sixth ribs at the midclavicular line. The surface projection of the lungs on the posterior chest is illustrated in *Figure 5-5*. The apices of the lungs extend to the first thoracic vertebra; the lower borders vary with respiration. On inspiration, the lung border drops to about $T_{12}$, and on exhalation it rises to about $T_{10}$. As projected onto the right lateral chest wall, the right *horizontal fissure* separating the upper and middle lobes of the right lung runs from a point slightly posterior to the midaxillary line at the fifth rib horizontally to the fourth costochondral junction *(Figure 5-6)*. The right *oblique fissure*, which separates the right upper and middle lobes from the lower lobe, extends from the fourth thoracic vertebra posteriorly and extends laterally and downward to cross the fifth rib at the midaxillary line. It continues anteriorly to the junction of the sixth rib and the midclavicular line. The left oblique fissure (separating the left upper and lower lobes) projects onto the left lateral chest

84

wall in the same manner as the right oblique fissure projects onto the right lateral chest wall *(Figure 5-7)*. As projected onto the left lateral chest wall, the left oblique fissure extends from the fourth thoracic vertebra posteriorly, to the sixth costochondral junction, crossing the fifth rib at the midclavicular line.

In *Figure 5-8* it can be seen that the projection of the lungs and lobar anatomy onto the anterior chest wall is comprised predominantly of the upper and middle lobes on the right and the upper lobe on the left; very little of the lower lobes can be identified on the anterior chest. However, most of the projection of the lungs and lobar anatomy on the posterior thorax is occupied by the lower lobes; the remainder is occupied by the upper lobes *(Figure 5-5)*.

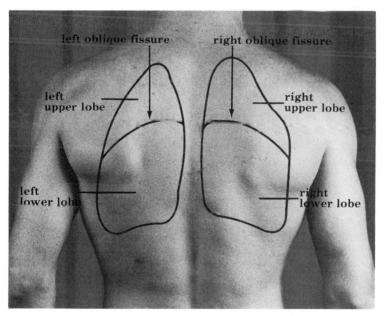

**Figure 5-5.** Surface projection of the lungs and lobar anatomy on the posterior chest wall.

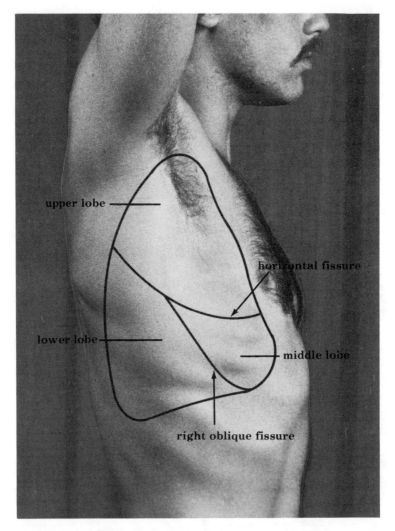

*Figure 5-6.* Surface projection of the right lung (including lobar anatomy) on the right lateral chest wall.

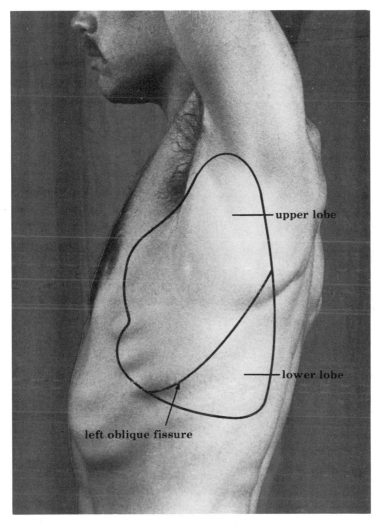

***Figure 5-7.*** Surface projection of the left lung (including lobar anatomy) on the left lateral chest wall.

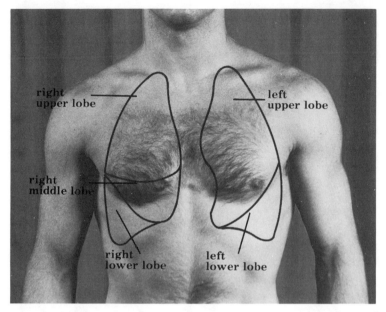

**Figure 5-8.** Lung borders including lobar anatomy on anterior chest wall. Note lung margins extend above clavicle on both sides.

## Segmental Anatomy of the Lungs

A knowledge of the segmental anatomy of the lungs is very important to the clinician who sees pulmonary patients routinely. This information is valuable not only to the clinician participating in bronchoscopies but also for proper patient positioning in chest physiotherapy and chest roentgenogram interpretation. The right lung is comprised of three lobes: an upper, a middle, and a lower lobe. The left lung has only two lobes: an upper lobe and a lower lobe. The lingular division of the left upper lobe, which is the lower division of the left upper lobe, corresponds to the right middle lobe. Table 5-2 lists the 18 bronchopulmonary segments which comprise the right and left lungs. The only differences in the segmental anatomy of the two lungs are: 1) the upper division of the left upper lobe, which corresponds to the right upper lobe, has only two segments, whereas the right upper lobe has three segments, and 2) the left lower lobe is considered to have only four segments, whereas the right lower lobe has five segments (Fraser, 1977; Jackson, 1943); on the left side, the medial basal bronchus is actually a branch of the left anterior basal and not a separate branch of the main lower lobe bronchus.

**Table 5-2. Bronchopulmonary segments.**

| Right Lung | |
|---|---|
| **upper lobe:** | apical<br>posterior<br>anterior |
| **middle lobe:** | lateral<br>medial |
| **lower lobe:** | superior<br>medial basal<br>anterior basal<br>lateral basal<br>posterior basal |

| Left Lung | | |
|---|---|---|
| **upper lobe:** | upper division: | apical posterior<br>anterior |
| | lower (lingular)<br>division: | superior<br>inferior |
| **lower lobe:** | superior<br>anteromedial basal<br>lateral basal<br>posterior basal | |

## Inspection of the Chest

Inspection of the chest is valuable in the assessment of chest symmetry, thoracic configuration, and the pattern of respiration. For optimal results, again the room should be well-lighted and the patient should be in an upright position. The male patient should be stripped to the waist, and the female patient should be provided with a gown which allows access to the anterior and posterior chest.

Generally, the first thing the examiner notices when inspecting the chest is chest symmetry. It should be remembered that no anatomical structure or area is perfectly symmetrical, and the thorax is no exception. For example, if the patient has used one arm considerably more than the other arm, there will probably be greater muscle development on one side. The clavicles should protrude equally and are more prominent in men than in women. The anteroposterior (AP) diameter of the chest in the normal adult is less than the transverse diameter; however, the AP diameter will gradually increase with age and will be greatly increased in patients with chronic obstructive pulmonary disease. With experience, one will learn to be able to tell whether the size and shape of the chest is normal for a given patient.

Another aspect of the thorax to notice is the general slope of the ribs. The width of the *costal angle* (the angle formed by the intersection of the two costal borders) should be less than 90° *(Figure 5-2)*. This angle normally widens during inspiration, but in patients with chronic emphysema, it remains wide during all phases of respiration.

### Thoracic Deformities

It is important for the clinician to be able to detect any alterations in the normal shape of the thoracic cage. If there is any gross abnormality present, it is usually readily apparent. Two of the more common anterior chest wall deformities are *pectus carinatum* and *pectus excavatum*. Pectus carinatum, or pigeon breast, is present when the patient's sternum bulges forward, not unlike that of a bird *(Figure 5-9)*. In this congenital condition, the chest configuration can be altered dramatically; however, lung function is rarely compromised. Pectus excavatum, or funnel breast, is a congenital condition in which the lower part of the sternum is depressed posteriorly *(Figure 5-10)*. In severe cases, pectus excavatum can result in displacement of the heart to the point where cardiac function is adversely affected. A third and fairly common chest wall abnormality which occurs secondarily to chronic pulmonary emphysema is *barrel chest (Figure 5-11)*. The increased AP diameter of the chest in this condition results in a barrel-like configuration of the chest. The intercostal spaces are widened, the costal angle is increased, and the chest appears to be in a state of hyperexpansion.

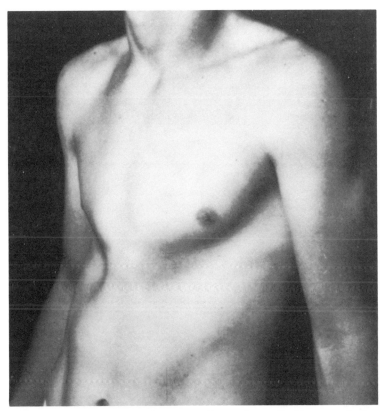

**Figure 5-9.** Pectus carinatum (pigeon breast). Sternum bulges outward. (From Ravitch, M.M., "Disorders of the chest wall" in *Davis-Christopher textbook of surgery, the biological basis of modern surgical practice,* 12th ed. Philadelphia: W.B. Saunders Co., 1981.)

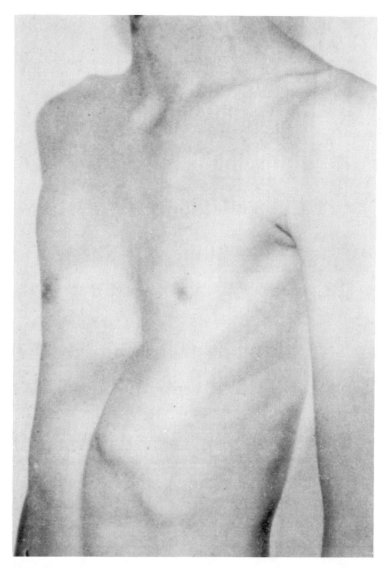

***Figure 5-10.*** Pectus excavatum (funnel breast). Note the inward depression of the sternum. (From Kampmeier, R.H., and T.M. Blake, *Physical examination in health and disease,* 4th ed. Philadelphia: F.A. Davis Co., 1970.)

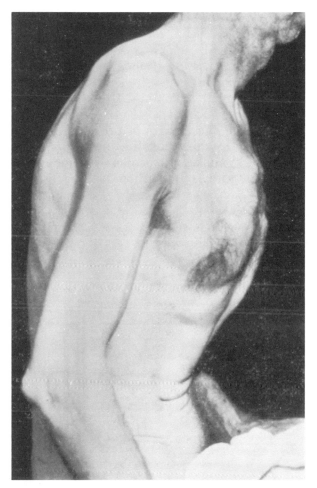

*Figure 5-11.* Barrel chest. The anteroposterior diameter is increased and appears to be in a state of permanent hyperinflation. There is also an increase in dorsal kyphosis. (From Kampmeier, R.H., and T.M. Blake, *Physical examination in health and disease,* 4th ed. Philadelphia: F.A. Davis Co., 1970.)

There are also several congenital spinal deformities that can severely affect the respiratory system. *Kyphosis (Figure 5-12)* is an exaggerated forward curvature of the thoracic spine. A smooth forward curve can be the result of poor posture, ankylosing spondylitis, or rheumatoid arthritis and is commonly associated with a barrel chest. The angular type of thoracic kyphosis involves a more acute curvature (gibbus) and can be due to a compression fracture of the vertebrae, tuberculosis, or malignancy. *Scoliosis (Figure 5-13)* is a spinal deformity in which there is an increased lateral curvature of the spine. Scoliosis usually consists of two curvatures: the original curve, and a compensatory curve in the opposite direction; combined, these two curves give the spine an S-shape. Scoliosis is usually due to neuro-muscular disease in the early years of life and ranges in severity from barely noticeable to debilitating. *Kyphoscoliosis,* a combination of kyphosis and scoliosis, is not uncommon and can also compromise the cardiopulmonary system.

Another type of spinal deformity is *lordosis (Figure 5-14)*, which is a disease of the lumbar spine and/or hips resulting in increased backward concavity of the lower back. This can be the result of compensation for a large abdomen during pregnancy, obesity, or one of the previously mentioned spinal deformities.

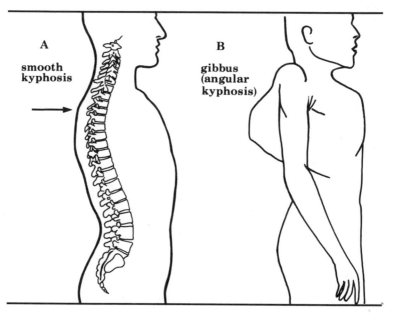

*Figure 5-12.* (**A**) Smooth kyphosis. The thoracic spine is curved by disease of several of the vertebrae. (**B**) Angular kyphosis. The angle or gibbus is formed by collapse of the body of a vertebra. The increased concavity of the spinal curve results in an increased anteroposterior diameter of the thorax.

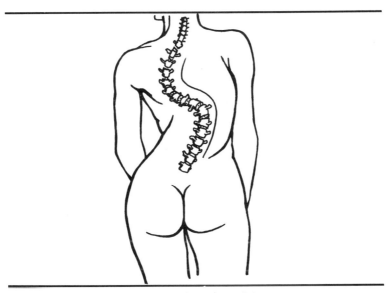

**Figure 5-13.** Scoliosis. An inclination of the thoracic spine to one side results in a compensatory displacement of the spine in the lumbar area, creating an S-curve.

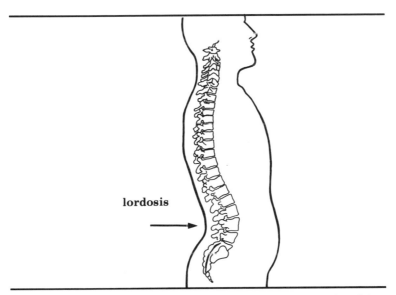

**Figure 5-14.** Lordosis, a disease of the lumbar spine and/or hips, results in increased backward concavity of the lumbar region. The thoracic spine is displaced posteriorly.

### *Retractions and Use of the Accessory Muscles of Inspiration*

The patient who is short of breath and has an increased work of breathing very often demonstrates retractions and use of the accessory muscles of inspiration. A retraction is a shortening of a muscle underneath the surface of the chest wall resulting in a drawing inward of that area of the chest with each breath. Retractions are caused by the patient's generation of a greater than normal negative force in an effort to get air into the lungs. They are commonly seen in the supraclavicular areas and the intercostal spaces. Infants, having more pliable thoracic cages than adults, often demonstrate sternal retractions in addition to supraclavicular and intercostal retractions.

Use of the accessory muscles of inspiration is also a sign of the patient's increased work of breathing. As mentioned, these muscles include the scalenes, the sternocleidomastoids, and the trapezius muscles *(Figure 5-15).*

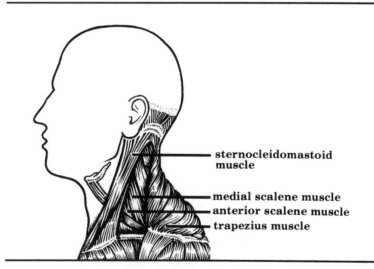

— sternocleidomastoid muscle

— medial scalene muscle
— anterior scalene muscle
— trapezius muscle

*Figure 5-15.* Accessory muscles of inspiration: scalenes, sternocleidomastoid and trapezius muscles.

The scalenes have as their origin the lower five cervical vertebrae and insert into the first and second ribs. Their importance in respiration lies in their elevation of the first two ribs. This helps to provide support for the apex of the lung, preventing it from herniating, which can occur in patients with a chronic cough. Because of their insertion, the scalenes are more active at larger lung volumes since it is then that the upper chest is more active in thoracic expansion.

The sternocleidomastoid muscles, one on each side of the neck, are probably the most important accessory muscles of inspiration. They originate at the manubrium and the clavicle and insert into the mastoid process and the occipital bone. The main action of these muscles is to elevate the sternum, which increases the anteroposterior diameter of the chest. Through this action, these muscles move the ribs upwards but not outwards. This accounts for the up-and-down movement of the chest with very little lateral expansion during inspiration, characteristic of patients with chronic obstructive pulmonary disease. In some patients, one sternocleidomastoid muscle may be shorter and more prominent than the other. This results in the head being tipped to one side, a condition called *torticollis* or wryneck *(Figure 5-16)*. If this condition is present but the muscles are not prominent, have the patient straighten the head; one muscle will tense more than the other.

The two trapezius muscles, one on each side of the neck and shoulders, are generally considered accessory muscles of inspiration because they extend the neck and facilitate the action of the sternocleidomastoids. The trapezius is active in some patients during quiet respiration. In the severely dyspneic patient, the trapezius can be seen to contract at the end of a maximal inspiration.

If the patient's work of breathing is increased, the accessory muscles of inspiration will come into action in a sequential fashion. If the work of breathing is mildly increased, the scalene muscles can be visualized; when the work of breathing is moderately increased, the sternocleidomastoid muscles are also active. When the work of breathing is severely increased, the activity of all three major accessory muscles of inspiration including the trapezius muscle can be appreciated.

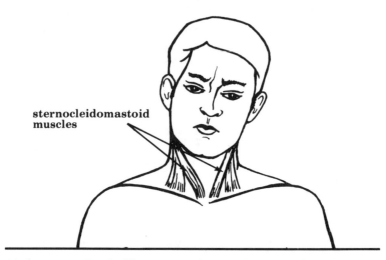

***Figure 5-16.*** Torticollis or wryneck, a condition resulting from one sternocleidomastoid muscle being shorter than the other. The shorter sternocleidomastoid causes the head to incline toward its side.

## Rate, Type, and Pattern of Breathing

While observing the patient, it is important to note the respiratory rate, the symmetry of the respirations, and the pattern of breathing. This can best be accomplished by having the patient sit upright while the examiner views from the front. In the normal adult at rest, the respiratory rate is between 14 and 20 breaths per minute. In the febrile patient, however, the respiratory rate can increase to about four additional cycles per minute for every °F above normal.

As air is drawn into the lungs due to changes in intrathoracic pressure, the diaphragm moves downward and the chest wall moves upward and outward. The lateral lower chest is the optimal area to visually assess thoracic expansion since most ventilation occurs here. In both men and women, the two sides of the thorax should move in synchrony. The respiratory activity in males tends to be predominantly diaphragmatic, while in females it is generally more costal. Sometimes asymmetrical chest movement is not as evident during quiet respiration as it is during forced respirations. Therefore, it is a good idea to evaluate chest excursion in both situations.

Because many conditions affect a patient's pattern of respiration, one should be able to recognize the commonly observed abnormalities in breathing. Some abnormal breathing patterns are indicative of pulmonary disorders, while others represent abnormal metabolic or central nervous system conditions.

A patient's subjective awareness of difficulty and effort in breathing is called *dyspnea*. Normally one is not aware of any work involved in breathing while at rest. Some patients complain of dyspnea only after exercise, which is not unusual; however, other patients become dyspneic after walking from their bed to the bathroom.

There are basically two types of dyspnea: inspiratory and expiratory. Inspiratory dyspnea usually occurs when there is an impediment to air flow in the upper airway, trachea, or large bronchi. This can be the result of foreign body aspiration, soft tissue obstruction, or tumor and is manifested by a high-pitched, crowing sound heard during inspiration called *stridor*. Also, the use of the accessory muscles of inspiration and/or retractions can be seen in the patient with inspiratory dyspnea.

Expiratory dyspnea implies an obstruction to the outflow of air from the lungs and involves the smaller airways. This type of dyspnea is commonly seen in patients with chronic obstructive pulmonary disease and is characterized by expiratory wheezing and a subsequent prolonged expiratory time.

*Tachypnea* is a respiratory rate faster than normal, whereas *bradypnea* is a respiratory rate slower than normal. An increase in the depth of respiration is called *hyperpnea*. Shallow respiration is called *hypopnea*.

Metabolic conditions resulting in acidosis elicit a compensatory response by the respiratory system. Diabetic ketoacidosis, renal failure, or drugs causing metabolic acidosis will cause a pattern of deep, regular, and often rapid respiration called *Kussmaul breathing (Figure 5-17)*. One of the most common forms of periodic breathing is *Cheyne-Stokes respiration*. This pattern of breathing is related to the medulla's diminished sensitivity to carbon dioxide tensions or to afferent stimuli (Delp, 1975). Cheyne-Stokes respiration can be the result of meningitis, cardiac disease, or brain tumors, among other etiologies. Cheyne-Stokes respiration is characterized by initially shallow breathing increasing gradually in depth to a point after which there is a gradual return to shallow breathing followed by a period of apnea *(Figure 5-17).* This period of apnea can last from five to forty seconds (Hopkins, 1965), after which this pattern of crescendo/decrescendo in the depth of respirations followed by apnea repeats itself. This type of respiratory activity is usually a sign of grave prognostication.

A variation of Cheyne-Stokes respiration is *Biot's breathing, (Figure 5-17),* in which there may be one or more breaths of varying depth followed by a period of apnea. This irregularity in breathing can be slow or rapid, shallow or deep, or any combination thereof. Biot's respiration is most commonly observed in patients with meningitis or other intracranial diseases.

*Sighing* occurs when the normal respiratory pattern is interrupted by a deep inspiration followed by a prolonged expiratory time. This pattern of breathing is rarely associated with organic disease and is usually seen in neurotic patients.

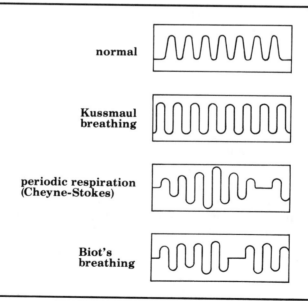

normal

Kussmaul breathing

periodic respiration (Cheyne-Stokes)

Biot's breathing

*Figure 5-17.* Patterns of respiration. Kussmaul breathing, Cheyne-Stokes respiration, and Biot's breathing compared to the normal ventilatory pattern.

# Palpation

## Chapter Six

## PALPATION

Palpation is the act of touching the patient with the hand in order to assess abnormalities of structure or movement. Because significant information concerning thoracic and extrathoracic abnormalities can be obtained by palpation, it is a useful adjunct to inspection. Palpation is performed in order to assess: 1) the skin and subcutaneous structures; 2) the trachea and other cervical structures; 3) thoracic expansion; 4) vocal fremitus; 5) crepitations; and 6) the point of maximal impulse (PMI).

## The Skin

Unless there are any specific lesions on the skin, palpation of the skin can be accomplished while evaluating the neck and chest. The level of general systemic hydration can be quickly ascertained by evaluating the skin *turgor,* which is the normal tension in the cells of the skin. This is assessed by pinching an area of the skin under which there is little subcutaneous fat, such as the back of the hand. This skin is pinched and then released, and should rapidly resume its usual configuration. If the patient is dehydrated, as is the case in many patients with chronic obstructive pulmonary disease, the skin fold will remain for several seconds after pinching, which indicates inadequate skin turgor.

## The Neck

Palpation of the neck should be done with the patient seated upright, relaxed, and looking directly forward. While the head and neck are in this position the laryngeal structures, thyroid gland, and trachea should be palpated.

### *Laryngeal Structures*

First, the *thyroid* cartilage (Adam's apple) should be identified. This is the largest cartilage of the larynx and is typically larger in men than in women in order to accommodate a larger larynx *(Figure 6-1).* Just below the thyroid cartilage is the cricoid cartilage. This cartilage serves as a useful landmark for identifying the thyroid gland which lies across the trachea just below the cricoid cartilages.

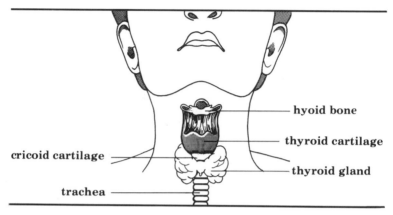

**Figure 6-1.** Normal neck anatomy. Anterior view of larynx including the hyoid bone, thyroid and cricoid cartilages, and thyroid gland.

### Thyroid Gland

Normally, the thyroid gland is not visible, but when hyperthrophy occurs, a fullness can be felt between the trachea and the sternocleidomastoid muscle. Its relative position can be seen in *Figure 6-1*. Palpation of the thyroid gland can be accomplished from either the front or the back. When examining the patient from the back, the examiner's fingers are placed adjacent to the trachea with the thumbs resting on the posterior neck *(Figure 6-2)*. As the patient swallows, the thyroid gland can be felt to move under the fingers. If the examiner chooses to palpate the thyroid gland from in front of the patient *(Figure 6-3)*, the thumb is placed against the side of the thyroid cartilage and lateral pressure is exerted toward the side of the thyroid gland being examined. The other thumb and fingers surround the sternocleidomastoid muscle under which the thyroid gland can be felt. Identifying the thyroid gland in the patient with a short, thick neck may be difficult with either technique.

The thyroid gland should be palpated for size, consistency, and the presence of any nodules. Enlargement of the thyroid gland suggests the presence of a thyroid disease such as goiter or iodine deficiency.

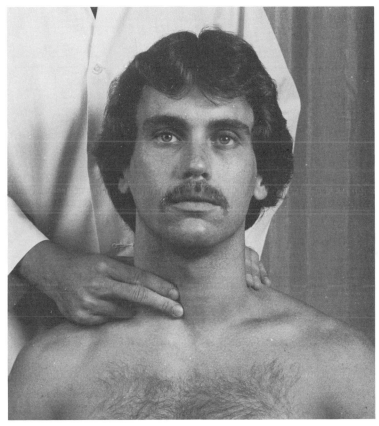

*Figure 6-2.* Palpation of thyroid gland from posterior position. The fingers are placed adjacent to the trachea with thumb resting on the posterior neck.

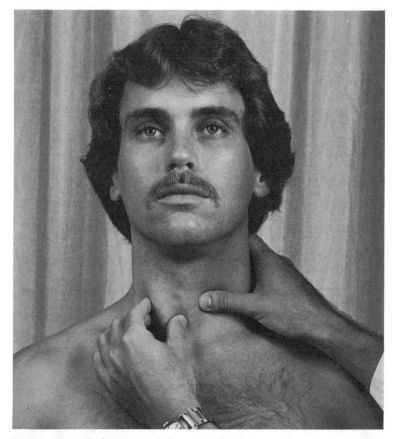

***Figure 6-3.*** Palpation of thyroid gland from anterior position. Thumb is placed against thyroid cartilage while other thumb and fingers surround sternocleidomastoid muscle. Thyroid gland can be felt under muscle.

## *Trachea*

Traditionally, tracheal palpation has been limited to rough evaluation of tracheal deviation. But the trachea should also be palpated for evidence of tracheal tug. Tracheal tug is most easily detected by having the patient elevate the chin, thereby tightening the trachea. Proper tension on the trachea is important; the tension on the trachea may be changed by asking the patient to lower or raise the chin. The examiner then places the tips of the thumb and index finger just below the cricoid cartilage and exerts a slight pressure upward. When tracheal tug is present, a definite pull coinciding with cardiac systole is felt which usually indicates the presence of an aortic aneurysm.

Lateral deviation of the trachea is an important clue to the presence of pulmonary or mediastinal disease and is best ascertained by palpating the tracheosternomastoid space (Rabin, 1965). This procedure involves placing the index finger in the space between the sternocleidomastoid muscle and the trachea to estimate the distance between these two structures *(Figure 6-4)*. Comparison of the width of this space on each side of the trachea will provide a good idea whether there is any tracheal deviation. The sternocleidomastoid space is narrowed on the side toward which the trachea is shifted. Some conditions will push the trachea to one side while other conditions will pull the trachea to one side. A list of the more common causes of tracheal deviation are found in Table 6-1. In the cases of bronchial obstruction and pneumothorax, palpation of the tracheosternomastoid space on inspiration and expiration is particularly useful. In both conditions, the trachea will move toward the side of the lesion during a deep inspiration and toward the opposite side during expiration.

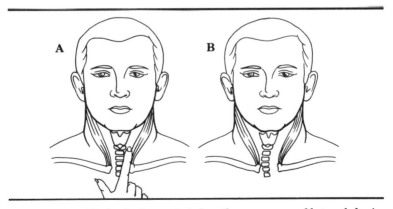

*Figure 6-4.* Method of ascertaining the presence of lateral deviation of the trachea. (**A**) On both sides of the trachea, the index finger is placed between the trachea and the sternocleidomastoid muscle and the distance between these two structures (the size of the tracheosternomastoid space) is estimated in order to compare the sizes of the two tracheomastoid spaces; in the healthy patient these will be equal. (**B**) Deviation of the trachea to the patient's right.

**Table 6-1. Causes of tracheal deviation.**

| Trachea deviated away from affected side | Trachea deviated toward affected side |
| --- | --- |
| tension pneumothorax | massive atelectasis |
| massive pleural effusion | phrenic nerve paralysis |
| mediastinal tumor | pneumonectomy |
| thyroid enlargement | |

## Thorax and Lungs

Palpation of the chest can provide considerable information regarding the presence of disease in the thorax and lungs. It can help diagnose breast masses, asymmetrical ventilation or the presence of space-occupying lesions in the chest. For optimal results from palpation, the entire chest should be exposed. In female patients, a gown can be arranged to permit access to the posterior thorax, lateral chest walls, and the anterior chest.

### *Thoracic Expansion*

One of the first things which should be evaluated in palpation of the chest is thoracic expansion. There are situations in which comparing the expansion of one hemithorax to the other is better accomplished by palpation than by simple inspection. Thoracic expansion can be assessed on the posterior or anterior chest. Posteriorly, one's hands should be placed over the lower ribs with the fingers spread slightly and extended. The hands are drawn medially, pulling the skin with them until the thumbs meet over the spinous processes of the vertebrae *(Figure 6-5)*. During quiet and deep respiration, the examiner should notice the divergence of the thumbs on inspiration, comparing the movement of both hands. Both hands should move an equal distance. Anteriorly, the examiner's hands should be placed over the lower ribs with the fingers extended toward the axillae. The skin is pulled medially until the thumbs meet at the midsternal line. The hands are then allowed to follow the chest movement during quiet and deep respiration while comparing the movement of both hands *(Figure 6-6)*. Again, both hands should move an equal distance during inspiration. Conditions such as pulmonary fibrosis, emphysema, pleural effusion, or fractured ribs will limit thoracic expansion over the involved area.

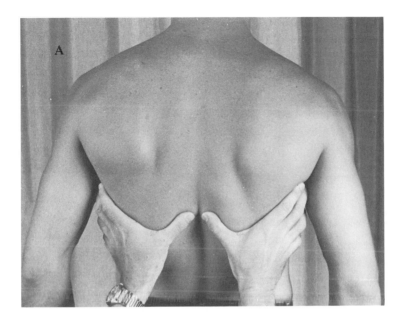

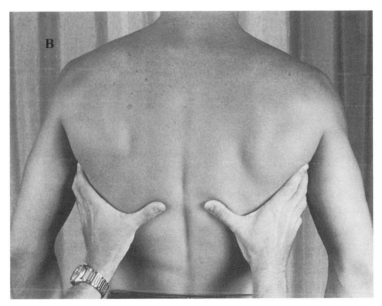

*Figure 6-5.* Technique of determining thoracic expansion of posterior chest. (**A**) Initial hand placement during rest or complete exhalation. (**B**) Both hands move an equal distance during inspiration.

109

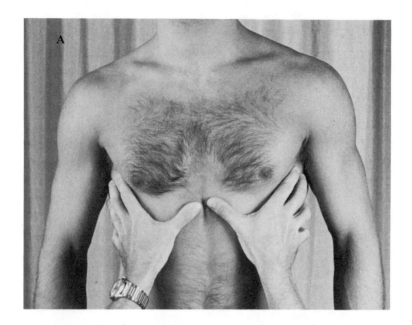

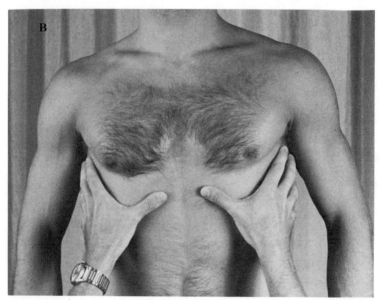

***Figure 6-6.*** Technique of determining thoracic expansion of anterior chest. (**A**) Initial hand placement during rest or complete exhalation. (**B**) Both hands move an equal distance during inspiration.

### *Vocal (tactile) Fremitus*

Fremitus is a vibration and vocal fremitus is a palpable vibration felt through the chest wall as the patient speaks. During phonation, the sounds produced are transmitted throughout the tracheobronchial tree causing the chest wall to vibrate. These vibrations can be felt by the hand; hence, the alternate term *tactile* fremitus.

To evaluate vocal fremitus, the patient is asked to say "ninety-nine, ninety-nine" or repeat "one, two, three" in as deep a voice as possible since lower frequencies produce greater vibrations. It is equally important that the patient speak with the same intensity or loudness each time, so the examiner can compare more accurately the vibrations in different areas of the chest. To feel the vibrations the ulnar surface of the hand or the palmar aspect of the finger tips is used. Some clinicians prefer to use both hands simultaneously, but if only one hand is used, corresponding areas of the thorax should be compared by moving from the apices to the bases *(Figure 6-7)*. It is important to remember that all areas of the chest should be palpated: anterior chest, posterior chest, and the right and left lateral thoracic areas.

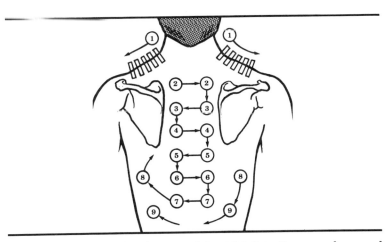

***Figure 6-7.*** In evaluating vocal (tactile) fremitus, numbers and arrows indicate sequence of examination on a posterior chest. The same sequence is used on an anterior chest. To evaluate the lateral thoracic areas, palpate just below the axilla, first on one side, then on the other. Then palpate the mid-lateral thoracic area on each side. Then palpate the lower thoracic area on each side.

Several factors affect the degree to which vocal fremitus can be felt, including the intensity of the voice, the pitch of the voice, the relationship of the bronchi to the chest wall, and the thickness of the chest wall (Prior, 1977). For example, if the patient's voice is too feeble, sufficient vibrations will not be palpable on the chest wall. Since the pitch of the female voice is high, fremitus may be diminished or even absent. Generally, fremitus is more intense over areas of the chest where the bronchi are closest to the chest wall. In the normal individual, fremitus is at its maximum intensity over the apices, particularly over the right upper lobe since this lobar bronchus comes off the trachea higher up than the left upper lobe bronchus. Conversely, fremitus is generally less intense at the bases.

In pathological conditions, vocal fremitus can be either increased or decreased. There will be increased vocal fremitus in conditions which favor the transmission of voice vibrations to the chest wall. This occurs when the ratio of lung tissue or solid or liquid matter to air is increased (Hopkins, 1965). Decreased fremitus will occur in conditions which interfere with the transmission of voice vibrations to the chest wall. Some of the more common causes of abnormal vocal fremitus are listed in Table 6-2.

**Table 6-2. Causes of abnormal vocal (tactile) fremitus.**

| Increased | Decreased |
|---|---|
| atelectasis | pneumothorax |
| pulmonary fibrosis | obstructed bronchus |
| pneumonia | pleural effusion |
| lung tumor | emphysema |
| pulmonary infarction | pneumonectomy |

### Crepitations

Subcutaneous crepitations can be felt when there are small air bubbles just under the skin. Sometimes called *subcutaneous emphysema,* this condition exists when air has escaped from lungs, intrapleural spaces, or mediastinum into the overlying tissues. When affected areas of skin are palpated a spongy crackling sensation can be felt. Crepitations can develop as a result of a pneumothorax, neck surgery (such as a tracheotomy), fractured ribs, or non-surgical penetrating wounds. Depending on the cause, crepitations are commonly felt in the supraclavicular areas of the neck, the axillae, and along the lateral aspects of the chest wall. Whenever subcutaneous crepitations are palpated, the etiology should always be sought.

### Point of Maximal Impulse (PMI)

When palpating the anterior thorax, the apical pulse or the *point of maximal impulse* (PMI) can be felt. This is the impulse at the apex of the heart that is caused by the force of the left ventricle against the chest wall during systole. Normally, the PMI is located in the fifth intercostal space just medial to the left midclavicular line. However, the PMI will vary with respiration and changes of position. If the patient takes in a deep breath and holds it, the PMI will move downward to the sixth intercostal space (Delp, 1975). Also, the point of maximal impulse will move to the right when the patient lies on the right side and to the left when the patient lies on the left side. If the patient has a severe pectus excavatum, the heart will be shifted to the left, thereby altering the position of the PMI. The clinician should not panic if the PMI is not exactly where it is expected.

# Percussion

*Chapter Seven*

## PERCUSSION

Percussion, as it is applied to clinical medicine, is the technique of striking the surface of the body and interpreting the character of the audible and palpable vibrations. The basic purpose of percussing the thorax is to determine the relative amount of air in the underlying structure, and, in order for percussion to be useful, the examiner must have a fundamental knowledge of anatomy. *Figure 7-1* shows the relationship of some internal organs to the chest wall. Abnormalities more than 5 cm from the chest wall or less than 2-3 cm in diameter cannot be detected by percussion (Delp, 1975). The technique can, however, easily detect shifts of organ boundaries and changes in the relative amounts of air, liquid, or solid material in the thorax.

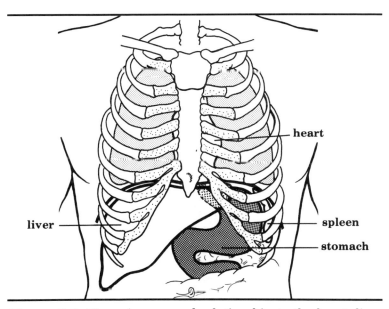

**Figure 7-1.** Thoracic cage and relationship to the heart, liver, stomach and spleen.

## Techniques of Percussion

There are basically two techniques of percussion. *Immediate* or *direct* percussion involves striking the chest wall directly with the tip of one or two fingers. However, since this method cannot detect smaller underlying lesions, it is not widely used. *Mediate* or *indirect* percussion involves striking an object held against the area to be examined on the chest wall. In this technique *(Figure 7-2)*, the distal joint of the middle finger of the left hand (if the examiner is right-handed) is placed firmly against the chest wall parallel to the ribs. The other fingers and palm are held *off* the skin. A quick blow is struck with the tip of the middle finger of the right hand against the distal joint of the middle finger of the left hand where it is pressed against the skin. The blows should be sharp, with immediate recoil of the striking finger.

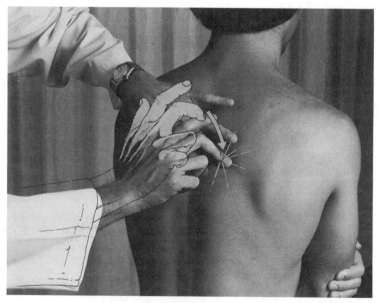

**Figure 7-2.** Technique of mediate (indirect) percussion. The distal joint of the middle finger of the left hand is placed firmly against the chest wall parallel to the ribs, and a quick, sharp blow is delivered to the distal joint with the tip of the middle finger of the right hand.

If the two fingers remain in contact too long, the sound may be dampened. A common mistake of beginners is to percuss from the elbow. For best results, the striking finger should be slightly flexed and the forearm should be held stationary with the movement occuring at the wrist. The amount of force required to produce a percussion sound is directly proportional to the thickness of the thorax. A muscular or obese patient will require a greater percussing force than a thin individual. As one develops the technique of percussion, it is important to become sensitive to the vibrations received from the chest wall by the finger in contact with the patient. In some cases, the perceived vibrations can be at least as informative as the sound of the percussion note.

The patient should be in the supine position when percussing the anterior chest. To evaluate the lateral and posterior chest wall, have the patient straddle a chair and lean forward against the back of the chair with the shoulders rotated forward. This will project the scapulae out of the field of evaluation. The recommended sequence for percussing the anterior and posterior chest is shown in *Figure 7-3.*

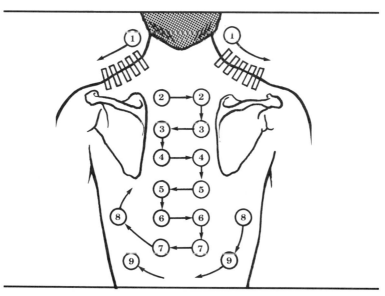

*Figure 7-3.* Sequence and pattern of percussion on posterior chest as indicated by the numbers and arrows. Anterior chest is percussed in the same sequence.

119

## Characteristics of Percussion Notes

As the chest is percussed, underlying structures such as the thoracic wall and the lungs begin to vibrate. Each vibration produces a characteristic sound wave, and different structures will produce different percussion notes depending on the amount of air within the underlying area. To better interpret the various percussion notes, one should have an understanding of the factors that characterize sound waves.

### Pitch

The pitch (or frequency) of a sound wave is determined by the number of vibrations per second that are emitted. The greater the number of vibrations, the higher the pitch. In contrast, fewer vibrations produce a lower pitch. It is difficult to place the pitch of percussion notes on the musical scale because they more closely resemble noises rather than musical tones. However, a relative pitch can be determined when compared to the pitch of other percussion notes.

### Intensity

The intensity (or amplitude) of a sound is the measure of the loudness or softness of the tone. A loud sound has a greater intensity than a soft sound. The intensity of a percussion note is influenced by two factors: 1) the type of substance through which the sound waves must pass before reaching the ear and 2) the force of percussion required to produce the sound. Because different tissues conduct sounds differently, the intensity of a note can help the examiner determine the type of tissue being percussed.

### Duration

The duration of a percussion note is the length of time for which the note is heard. This characteristic can be helpful because some percussion notes are heard longer than others.

### Quality

This characteristic is difficult to describe because it is a subjective interpretation based primarily on the overtones of the fundamental frequency of the percussion note. For example, the quality of a tone is what makes a note played on a piano sound different from the same note played on a guitar.

The quality of a sound resulting from percussion is important because it helps the examiner to distinguish sounds originating from different structures. Terms such as "hollow", "musical", or "thud-like" are utilized.

## Percussion Notes and Their Location

When percussion is performed, different notes can be heard depending on the amount of air in the underlying structures. An air-filled lung will sound different from the tone heard over a solid structure like the heart or liver. However, there is no "normal" percussion note. Depending on the thickness of the chest wall and the type of tissue being percussed, identical areas on the chests of two different patients can sound different. In any one individual, the percussion notes at the apex and base of the same lung can sound slightly different because of differences in the chest wall thickness and the volume of air under these areas. The following descriptions of the five types of percussion notes should provide help in interpreting percussion sounds over different areas of the chest.

### Resonant Percussion Note

A *resonant* percussion note generally is heard over "normal" lungs. It is relatively low in pitch and is long in duration. The resonant percussion note contains many overtones which give it a hollow quality, and resonance can be elicited on the right anterior hemithorax from the apex down to approximately the fifth rib. Below this level, however, the dome of the hemidiaphragm and the liver will produce a dull note. On the left side of the anterior thorax, a resonant note can be percussed from the apex down to the fourth or fifth intercostal space. In the normal individual, an area of dullness outlines the cardiac border extending a maximum of 7 or 8 cm left of the midsternal line (Kampmeier, 1970). Percussion over the sternum and the breasts of female patients has minimal value and should be avoided.

Posteriorly, resonant percussion should begin at the apices and outline two bands of resonance over the trapezius muscles. Each of these bands (Kronig's isthmus) is about 2-3 inches wide and is bordered medially by the neck muscles and laterally by the soft tissues of the shoulder *(Figure 7-4)*.

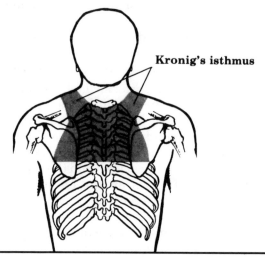

**Kronig's isthmus**

*Figure 7-4.* Kronig's isthmus. At the apices, two bands of resonance run over the shoulders like shoulder straps (shaded areas on illustration) and are known as Kronig's isthmus.

The posterior chest should be resonant to percussion down to the hemidiaphragms, which are about at the level of the tenth ribs.

### Hyperresonant Percussion Note

A *hyperresonant* percussion note is generally louder than a resonant note and has a "booming" quality. It is lower in pitch than a resonant note, quite long in duration, and creates a noticeable vibratory sensation. Hyperresonance can be heard in the adult with a thin chest wall on deep inspiration as well as in children. Pathologically, a hyperresonant note is the result of an increase in the amount of air in the thorax. This can be due to air-trapping in emphysema and during an asthmatic attack or a pneumothorax.

### Tympanic Percussion Note

The *tympanic* percussion note is probably the most distinctive tone of all five percussion sounds because of the absence of overtones. It also has the highest pitch of the percussion notes. The tympanic note is slightly louder than the resonant note and is only moderately long in duration. The fact that this sound is produced by air in an enclosed chamber, such as the stomach or intestines, gives it a "drum-like" quality. The greater the tension within the chamber, the higher the pitch. The tympanic note is not normally heard in the chest except below the left hemidiaphragm over the stomach bubble. Abnormalities which can cause a tympanic percussion note in the chest include large pulmonary cavities due to cancer or fungal diseases, and tension pneumothorax.

### *Dull Percussion Note*

A *dull* percussion note is heard when there is decreased air content in the underlying tissues. This tone is high-pitched, relatively soft in intensity, and shorter in duration than the resonant note. The dull note most closely resembles a "thud" when heard, and, because the underlying tissues producing this sound are not set into motion when percussed, very few vibrations are perceived by the finger in contact with the chest. Normally, dull percussion notes are heard over the liver, heart, diaphragm, spleen, and bony structures. The fact that the percussion note over these organs is noticeably different from that heard over the lungs can be used to determine the size of the heart, liver, and spleen. This fact also makes percussion useful in ascertaining diaphragmatic excursion.

An abnormality exists if a dull percussion note is heard over the area where the lungs should be. This occurs in conditions where solid or liquid material has replaced normally aerated lungs or when fluid or solid matter accumulate in the intrapleural space. For this reason, percussion is invaluable in determining the upper level of a pleural effusion. Generally, the same abnormal conditions resulting in an increased vocal fremitus will also result in dullness to percussion in this area. Table 7-1 lists some of the more common abnormal causes of a dull percussion note heard over the chest.

### *Flat Percussion Note*

The *flat* percussion note is actually a more extreme example of dullness. It can be heard over areas of the chest which are completely airless. This note is soft in intensity, high-pitched, and quite short in duration. The sound of a completely flat percussion note is no different than the sound of the impact of the percussing finger against the finger in contact with the patient. A flat note can be elicited when percussing the thigh. Examples of abnormal causes of a flat percussion note on the chest include a pneumonectomy and massive atelectasis. Table 7-2 summarizes the characteristics of the various percussion notes elicited on physical examination.

**Table 7-1. Pathological causes of a dull percussion note.**

atelectasis

lung tumors

pneumonia

pulmonary fibrosis

pulmonary edema

pleural effusion

pleural thickening

pleural tumors

## Diaphragmatic Excursion

Diaphragmatic mobility can be estimated by percussion on the posterior chest wall. Ideally, the patient should sit backwards on a chair, exposing the entire back, and should be instructed to take a deep breath and hold it. The clinician should then percuss down one side of the back in the midscapular line until the percussion note changes from resonant to dull. The examiner should note the level at which this change occurs. The patient is then instructed to exhale maximally and again hold the breath. Percussion is then repeated down the same side of the posterior chest until the lower margin of resonance is detected. This level is noted also. (This procedure should be performed rapidly to prevent the patient from becoming short of breath.) The entire procedure is then repeated for the other hemidiaphragm. The distance between the two marks *(Figure 7-5)* on each side of the back represents the range of motion of the diaphragm. Normally, diaphragmatic excursion is about 3-5

**Table 7-2. Characteristics of the normal percussion notes.**

| Note | Pitch | Intensity | Duration | Quality |
|---|---|---|---|---|
| Resonant | Low | Moderately loud | Long | Hollow |
| Hyperresonant | Very low | Very loud | Very long | Booming |
| Tympanic | High | Loud | Moderately long | Drum-like |
| Dullness | High | Moderately soft | Short | Thud |
| Flatness | High | Soft | Very short | Extremely dull |

125

centimeters on both sides. However, because the domes of the hemidiaphragms are 10-15 centimeters below the surface of the posterior chest wall, percussion can only approximate the degree of diaphragmatic excursion.

Certain abnormal conditions will alter diaphragmatic mobility. In the patient with severe emphysema, the diaphragm will be fixed in a low position. Conversely, the hemidiaphragms will be particularly high in the patient with ascites or one who is pregnant. Other restrictive disorders such as chest wall deformities and neuromuscular diseases will also result in a diminished range of diaphragmatic movement.

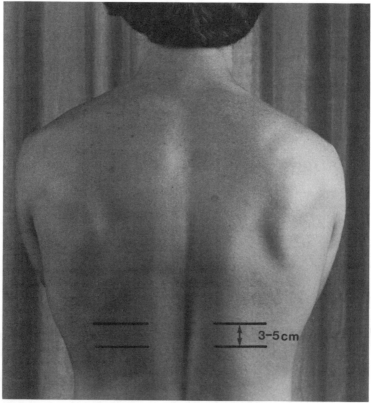

*Figure 7-5.* Estimating diaphragmatic mobility, or diaphragmatic excursion. The upper lines represent the level of hemidiaphragms after a complete expiration. Lower lines represent the level of the hemidiaphragms at the end of a maximal inspiration. The distance between the two marks normally is 3 to 5 cm.

# Auscultation

*Chapter Eight*

## AUSCULTATION

Auscultation is the process of listening for sounds produced within the body, and is done chiefly to ascertain the condition of the lungs, heart, abdomen, and other organs. It is also one of the most important of the physical examination techniques for the assessment of pulmonary disorders. Auscultation can be accomplished by either *immediate auscultation,* which consists of placing the ear directly against the chest wall, or by *mediate auscultation,* which is performed with the aid of a stethoscope interposed between the ear and the part of the body being examined. The latter method is almost universally employed.

### Auscultory Tones

Vibrations of a certain frequency range and intensity are produced and are perceived as sounds due to air moving through the tracheobronchial tree during respiration, and as a result of the contractile force of the heart. These sounds differ from one another in pitch, intensity, quality and duration, and because of this, sounds auscultated from the chest should be evaluated in respect to these differing characteristics.

As sound is transmitted to the chest wall, it is influenced by varying degrees of reflection that take place where there are changes in media, i.e., from the heart to the surrounding muscles. It is the density of these tissues that primarily determines the amount of sound reflection; part of the sound is reflected and part passes through to the surface of the chest wall. The human ear is most sensitive to frequencies in the range of 1,000-5,000 cycles per second. Since almost all of the sounds emitted from the chest are composed of frequencies below 1,000 cycles per second (Cabot, 1925), the unaided ear generally is not sensitive enough to make distinctions among different sounds. Because of this, a device is required to selectively filter and magnify chest sounds: the stethoscope.

## The Stethoscope

Ever since Laennec invented the stethoscope over 150 years ago, this instrument has epitomized the bedside clinician. The modern stethoscope consists of four basic parts: earpieces, tubing, a bell chest piece, and a diaphragm chest piece *(Figure 8-1)*.

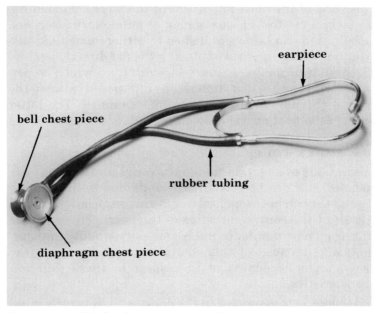

*Figure 8-1.* The basic parts of a stethoscope.

### *Earpieces*

The earpieces should fit the ear canal snugly without becoming uncomfortable after a few minutes of use. Proper fit of the earpieces is important because an enclosed pathway is essential for efficient transmission of sounds from the chest wall to the ear. Any leaks in this enclosed system not only admit extraneous noise, but also result in decreased transmission efficiency by destroying the acoustical seal. The earpieces should be examined periodically for cracks and cerumen or dirt accumulation which might interfere with auscultation.

### Stethoscope Tubing

An important consideration related to stethoscope performance is the length and caliber of the tubing. The tubing should be as short as possible for maximum efficiency but long enough to be convenient for the user. For the frequency range in which most chest sounds fall, tubing length exerts a significant effect. For example, as the tubing length increases, the efficiency of the stethoscope decreases. A length of approximately 10-12 inches (25-30 cm) satisfies requirements of efficiency and convenience. Longer tubing compromises the transmission of high-pitched sounds. The internal diameter of the tubing should be small, but must be large enough to prevent closure when the tubing is bent slightly. The internal caliber should be equal to that of the earpieces and the chest pieces. Commercial stethoscope tubing with a caliber of 3/16 inch is satisfactory. The wall of the tubing should be thick in order to minimize interference from external noise.

Debate continues about the practice of incorporating two separate tubes between the chest piece and the earpiece as opposed to a single tube leading from the chest piece to the earpiece. The single-tube models have been demonstrated to result in distortion at higher frequencies (Ertel, 1966). Therefore, despite their neat appearance and compactness, the single-tube stethoscopes are acoustically inferior to their double-tube counterparts.

### Chest Pieces

The two chest pieces commonly used are the bell and the diaphragm. The *bell* is a hollow cone usually made of plastic or metal. The bell, which should be about one inch in diameter to examine an adult's chest, transmits almost all sounds from within the chest, but is particularly helpful when listening to low-pitched heart sounds. It is also useful when listening to lung sounds between the ribs of the very thin patient because it has a smaller contact area than the diaphragm chest piece, so that a seal is more easily attained. When using the bell, it should be applied *lightly* to the patient's chest. If it is pressed too firmly against the chest, the skin under the bell will be stretched taut, and its natural period of oscillation will increase. This will result in an increased response of the stethoscope to high-frequency sounds and the filtering out of most of the low-frequency sounds, a result which is undesirable.

The *diaphragm chest piece* is used to auscultate high-frequency sounds in the chest. It is comprised of a shallow cup covered by a thin plastic material which attenuates low-frequency sounds, making the remaining high-frequency sounds seem amplified. The diaphragm used on the adult should be 1 to 1-1/2 inches in diameter. For optimal results, it should be *firmly* placed against the chest so that interfering, extraneous sounds are not heard. Because the diaphragm filters out lower-pitched heart and chest sounds, the higher-pitched sounds are more easily heard, thereby reducing the masking effect. Masking is the difficulty detecting certain sounds in the presence of other sounds, much the same as the difficulty encountered hearing a conversation in a noisy room. Table 8-1 identifies the various sounds which can be successfully auscultated with the bell and the diaphragm chest pieces; however, with all these acoustical characteristics of stethoscopes in mind, it should be remembered that the most important part of the total system is the cerebrating activity of the individual between the earpieces.

Table 8-1. Chest sounds auscultated with diaphragm chest piece and with bell chest piece.

| Diaphragm | Bell |
| --- | --- |
| all lung sounds | third heart sound |
| first heart sound | fourth heart sound |
| second heart sound | diastolic murmurs |
| murmur of aortic regurgitation | murmur of congenital pulmonary valve regurgitation |
| systolic clicks | |

## Technique of Auscultation

Proper auscultation of the chest requires that the patient be positioned properly and that the patient understand the correct method of breathing. The patient should be seated upright with the shoulders rotated forward in a relaxed manner. This will move the scapulae partially out of the field of auscultation. It is most convenient for the right-handed examiner to position the patient on the examiner's right. The patient should be instructed to breathe slightly deeper than normal with the mouth open. Sometimes it is helpful to demonstrate the proper breathing technique to the patient.

One should use a systematic approach to auscultation similar to that of percussion. A recommended procedure involves first listening to the apices, then moving down the lateral aspects of the thorax to the bases, remembering to compare corresponding areas on each side. Several ventilatory cycles should be heard at each stethoscope position. The chest piece used should be placed directly on the skin; a gown or shirt between the chest piece and the thorax can produce misleading sounds. In order to eliminate interfering noises, sufficient pressure should be exerted on the bell or diaphragm to maintain the acoustical seal.

## Errors in Auscultation

Before beginning a discussion of breath sounds, it might be beneficial to the clinician to be aware of some of the common sources of error in auscultation.

1. When listening to the chest, many beginners tend to hear too much rather than too little. One must learn to concentrate on one sound at a time and disregard other sounds. It can be quite confusing to try to hear the first heart sound, for example, while also thinking about the breath sounds in the background. The ability to pick out the desired sound from among a group of others requires listening to many chests.

2. The sound of chest hair rubbing against the diaphragm is often mistaken for an abnormal breath sound. In patients with hairy chests, it is difficult to avoid these sounds as the thorax expands during inspiration. These sounds can be minimized by wetting the hair on the chest prior to auscultation.

3. Auscultating the chest of a very nervous or cold individual can lead to error. The sounds produced as the result of the muscles twitching are often misinterpreted as abnormal lung sounds. In the patient who is shivering, the sounds are probably muscular in origin. If there is doubt whether the sounds heard originate from the lungs

or the muscles, ask the patient to cough. Sounds associated with muscle movement will not be affected by coughing. Be certain the patient is using only those muscles required for respiration when auscultating the chest.

4. If one side of the bell chest piece is elevated and not in complete contact with the thorax, the resulting soft, breezy sound can be confusing. This sound is similar to that heard when a sea shell is held next to the ear and can be eliminated by making sure the bell forms a complete seal with the skin. Another cause of this misleading sound is improper fit of the earpieces in the ear because the earpieces are reversed. Because of the oblique direction of the auditory canal in each ear, the earpieces should be angled slightly *forward* for proper alignment of the earpiece tips with the ear canal. This will result in an acoustical seal in the ears and will eliminate the distracting noise.

5. Breathing on the stethoscope tubing by either the examiner or the patient will result in an extraneous noise. This error can be eliminated by simply repositioning the stethoscope tubing.

6. A crack in the diaphragm chest piece can lead to erroneous interpretations of thoracic sounds. To prevent this, periodically examine the diaphragm to be sure it is intact.

## Normal Breath Sounds

Auscultation of the chest traditionally has been an easy way to obtain information regarding the status of the lungs. However, many clinicians feel that lung sounds are not as precise an evaluation tool as other laboratory procedures. Therefore, auscultation of the lungs has become simply a cursory procedure in many cases. Much of the recent neglect of auscultation is the result of inadequate understanding of the mechanism of production of these sounds and the confusing terminology used to describe what is heard. The following discussion is a summary of the mechanisms currently thought responsible for the various breath sounds, and suggested terminology to use when describing breath sounds.

When auscultating the lungs of a healthy individual, the sounds heard at any one point represent a combination of sounds originating in different areas of the chest. Breath sounds have a unique quality depending upon the area of the chest being examined. The quality of breath sounds is influenced by the intensity of the sounds and the distance of the chest piece from the origin of the sounds.

Breath sounds heard over the chest of the normal individual are thought to be generated by the turbulence in the large airways (Forgacs, 1971). This turbulent flow creates vibrations which are transmitted through the lungs to the chest wall. As the sound travels toward the lung periphery, some of the higher frequencies are filtered by the normal lung tissue. Essentially, the normal lung acts as a low-pass filter, meaning it preferentially permits passage of low-pitched sounds (Murphy, 1980). This gives the sounds heard over the periphery of the lung fields a relatively low-pitched, muffled rushing quality. This breath sound is often referred to as "vesicular," from the Latin word for small vessels; however, since this term implies the sounds heard over the normal peripheral lung originate in the alveoli, it is recommended that these sounds simply be called *normal breath sounds*. An aid to identifying these sounds is the fact that they have an inspiratory component which is heard as being louder and longer in duration than the expiratory component. It is important to realize, however, that the total expiratory time is actually longer than the time devoted to inspiration, but that the inspiration period sounds longer than the expiration period because much of the expiration sound is inaudible.

In contrast to the normal breath sounds heard over most of the lung fields, the sounds over the large airways are louder, higher in pitch, and have a hollow tubular quality. These sounds, often referred to as "bronchial" or "tracheal" breath sounds, are heard in the normal chest over the trachea and over the midsternal line in the upper chest, as well as on both sides of the sternum. On the posterior chest, the sounds are heard between the scapulae. These breath sounds are also considered normal breath sounds, but their quality is different because the airways under these areas are relatively closer to the chest wall. Since there is less normal lung tissue between the large airways and the chest piece, fewer of the high frequencies of the sounds are filtered. It is the filtering phenomenon that accounts for the differences in quality between the lung sounds heard over the periphery and those heard over the large airways. Normal peripheral lung sounds are essentially filtered large-airway sounds.

Listening carefully to the timing of the expiratory component will help distinguish the sounds heard over the large airways just under the sternum from those sounds originating from the smaller airways heard over the majority of the chest. Sounds heard over the large airways have a longer expiratory phase than the breath sounds from the smaller airways. Also, there is a brief, silent pause between inspiration and expiration when listening to the large airways under the sternum and between the scapula.

In summary, lung sounds heard over the normal chest are all normal breath sounds; however, sounds heard over the large airways have a different quality than the sounds heard away from these large airways. The generating mechanisms are believed to be the same in both locations, but the filtering action of the lung tissue changes the quality of the sounds. It is recommended that the clinician auscultate as many normal chests as possible, so identification of the two normal qualities of breath sounds will be easier.

## Abnormal Breath Sounds

The description of abnormal breath sounds is a medical area where there is much ambiguity and confusion in terminology. Some clinicians go to great lengths to describe an abnormal sound in such meticulous detail that anyone outside that particular hospital would have difficulty recognizing the description. On the other extreme, some clinicians describe all abnormal lung sounds using the same term, which encourages a multitude of interpretations. In this discussion, a system of terminology is suggested which hopefully is succinct yet specific enough to adequately describe the abnormal breath sound.

The presence of decreased or absent breath sounds should be considered abnormal. If, after determining the stethoscope is functioning properly, breath sounds cannot be heard, one can assume there is either no aerated lung under the area being examined, or there is an intrapleural process blocking the transmission of sounds.

136

The absence of breath sounds caused by a loss of ventilation to all or part of the lung can be the result of upper or lower airway obstruction. Some common examples of airway obstruction include: foreign body aspiration, endobronchial tumors, laryngospasm, laryngeal edema, and a mucus plug obstructing a bronchus — all of which can result in decreased or even absent breath sounds. An endotracheal tube inserted too far into the airway causing it to cannulate the right mainstem bronchus can result in absent breath sounds over the left lung. Also, the surgical removal of lung tissue, as in a lobectomy or pneumonectomy, will result in absent breath sounds over the involved area.

Pleural abnormalities can also be the cause of absent breath sounds. The accumulation of air or fluid in the intrapleural space inhibits the transmission of breath sounds from the lungs to the chest wall. A pneumothorax or a pleural effusion can be responsible for absent breath sounds by creating a restriction to ventilation, and by blocking the sound vibrations before they reach the stethoscope. A summary of the common causes of absent breath sounds is found in Table 8-2.

**Table 8-2. Causes of absent breath sounds.**

| |
|---|
| Complete airway obstruction |
| Pneumothorax |
| Pleural effusion |
| Pneumonectomy |
| Massive obesity |
| Malposition of endotracheal tube |
| Atelectasis |

When the lung sounds heard over the large airways ("bronchial" breath sounds) are heard over the peripheral lung, this should be regarded as an abnormal breath sound. This will occur when there is an increase in lung tissue density (consolidation). When a consolidation of lung tissue exists, the filtering effect of the lung is diminished, allowing the higher-frequency sounds to be heard more clearly. There-

137

fore, breath sounds over the periphery will be similar to those over the large airways.

### Adventitious Sounds

Adventitious lung sounds are sounds not normally heard when auscultating the chest. They are not different classifications of the fundamental breath sounds, but rather are abnormal sounds superimposed on normal breath sounds. Adventitious sounds can be generally classified as either discontinuous or continuous sounds.

Discontinuous sounds are short, discrete, non-musical sounds heard in addition to the underlying breath sound. They have a range of frequencies from about 200 to 2,000 cycles per second, and their pitch may be either high or low depending upon which frequencies predominate. These discontinuous sounds have a "crackling" quality; hence the recommended term *crackles*. Forgacs (1967) suggested that crackles are generated by the explosive reopening of closed airways due to the development of a critical transmural pressure during inspiration. Other research (Nath, 1974) has confirmed this hypothesis. Crackles are predominantly inspiratory sounds and are rarely heard on expiration. The timing of inspiratory crackles has been correlated with their source. Early inspiratory crackles are believed to originate in the proximal and larger airways and are heard in patients with severe airway obstruction such as asthma, chronic bronchitis, and emphysema. Late inspiratory crackles arise from peripheral airways, each crackle representing the opening of an individual airway. The opening pressure developed later in inspiration is responsible for the delay in the sound being heard. Late inspiratory crackles are more common in restrictive lung disorders such as fibrosis, pneumonia, sarcoidosis, and edema secondary to congestive heart failure. Crackles are generally better heard at the lung bases and are not altered by coughing.

Crackles have been a central part of the confusion in lung sound terminology for many years. These sounds were originally described by the French physician Laennec as "rales" which is the French word for rattle. He chose this word to describe all adventitious sounds. To spare his patients the unpleasant feelings associated with this word, he used the Latin synonym "rhonchus" at the bedside. This was later translated by English writers to "wheeze". Since that time, many clinicians have coined very imaginative descriptions for rales such as "fine", "moist", "dry", and "velcro" rales. None of these terms has been acoustically defined; nevertheless, this inexact terminology is widespread.

Continuous adventitious sounds are longer in duration and musical in comparison to crackles and are referred to as *wheezes*. Wheezes are classified as either high-pitched or low-pitched depending upon the predominant frequencies heard. Historically, a low-pitched wheeze was known as a rhonchus and the high-pitched, continuous sound was referred to as a wheeze. The mechanism which produces both of these sounds is identical: vibrations are generated in the walls of narrowed or compressed airways as the air passes through at high velocities (Forgacs, 1967). The airways can be narrowed as a result of bronchoconstriction, edema, or mucous secretions. (A more detailed description of the production of wheezes can be found in Chapter 2.) The difference in character between high-pitched and low-pitched wheezes is the result of the filtering action of the lung. Since these sounds are produced by the same mechanism, it is unnecessary to distinguish between wheezes and rhonchi.

Another type of adventitious sound is the pleural friction rub. Normally the parietal and visceral pleural surfaces are smooth and quietly glide over one another during respiration. When one or both pleurae become inflamed and roughened, as the result of pleurisy, infection, or pulmonary infarction, a friction rub will result when the pleural surfaces rub together. The pleural friction rub has a grating or scraping quality, and sounds much the same as rubbing the thumb and index finger together next to one's ear. Although the friction rub can be heard during both phases of respiration, it is most commonly heard during inspiration, particularly near end-inspiration. Friction rubs are usually heard over the lateral and anterolateral aspects of the chest since this is the area of greatest thoracic excursion.

## Voice Sounds

When the examiner auscultates the chest of a normal individual as that person speaks, the voice sounds are blurred and indistinct. This occurs because many of the voice sounds are filtered before they reach the stethoscope. This voice sound heard over the normal lung is called *vocal resonance*. To elicit vocal resonance, the patient is asked to say "ninety-nine" or "one, two, three". Vocal resonance is produced by the same mechanism which produces tactile fremitus and will be increased or decreased by the same pathologic processes. There are three types of abnormal voice sounds which can be heard as the result of thoracic abnormalities.

1. **Bronchophony.** This denotes an increased clarity of the spoken word. As one auscultates the chest, the words sound louder than the normal vocal resonance. Individual syllables are not distinguishable, but the words are more distinct. Bronchophony can be heard in areas of the chest where previously normal alveoli are filled with fluid or replaced by compressed lung tissue. This occurs because of the principle that a liquid or solid medium transmits sounds better than an air-filled medium. Bronchophony is usually associated with the same disorders that produce an increased tactile fremitus and dullness to percussion, namely a consolidation, atelectasis, or partial compression of a bronchus by a tumor, among others.

2. **Whispered pectoriloquy.** This is the increased transmission of the whispered word to the chest wall. Normally, whispered sounds are heard very faintly and indistinctly over most of the chest. If whispered pectoriloquy is present, the whispered "one, two, three" or "ninety-nine" will be heard without difficulty as if the syllables were whispered directly into the stethoscope. Pectoriloquy will be present in the same conditions that produce bronchophony and is often heard before other abnormal lung sounds.

3. **Egophony.** Originally described by Laennec as a "goat voice", egophony is a modified form of bronchophony; the intensity is increased and the quality resembles a nasal sound. This sound can be imitated by speaking while closing the nostrils with the fingers. The sound can be elicited by having the patient say "E". If egophony is present, this "E" will sound like a nasal "A". Egophony is heard most often just above the upper level of a pleural effusion of moderate size. It can be clinically helpful in differentiating a pleural effusion from a consolidation.

140

## Heart Sounds

A description of chest auscultation would not be complete without a brief discussion of heart sounds. For proper cardiac auscultation, a quiet room is essential. It is equally important for the examiner to listen to specific parts of the cardiac cycle, which will facilitate identification of the individual heart sounds. Also, the examiner should use a stethoscope that has both a diaphragm and bell chest piece so that all four heart sounds can be heard more easily.

As with auscultation of lung sounds, the patient should be relaxed, comfortable, and either disrobed from the waist up or properly gowned. Thorough cardiac auscultation involves listening to the chest while the patient is in the sitting, supine, and left lateral decubitus positions.

### *First Heart Sound*

The first heart sound results from the closure of the atrioventricular valves (mitral and tricuspid). This sound occurs with the onset of the apical pulse and corresponds with ventricular systole. Since the first heart sound is a composite resulting from the closure of both the mitral and tricuspid valves, it has two components. Usually the closure of the mitral valve precedes the closure of the tricuspid valve, and distinguishing the two components is quite difficult in the normal individual. In patients with right bundle branch block, wide splitting of the mitral and tricuspid components of the first heart sound can be best heard by listening at the lower left sternal edge with a rigid diaphragm.

The intensity of the first heart sound is mainly influenced by the position of the cusps at the onset of ventricular contraction. If the valve cusps are wide apart due to continued blood flow from the atria to the ventricles, the first sound will probably be loud. The first sound will be diminished in conditions which interfere with sound transmission such as a pleural or pericardial effusion, emphysema, and obesity.

### *Second Heart Sound*

The second heart sound is produced by the closure of the semilunar valves. Like the first heart sound, the second sound is a composite sound resulting from the closure of the aortic and pulmonary valves. Normally, the aortic component precedes the pulmonary component. Distinguishing these two components is more easily accomplished than isolating the components of the first heart sound. The second sound normally splits at the end of normal inspiration and can best be heard in the second left intercostal space near the sternal border. The splitting of the second heart sound is due to the fact that an increase in ventricular stroke volume causes delay in valve closure. During inspiration, negative intrathoracic pressure is generated, which increases the venous return to the right side of the heart. This results in a greater stroke volume of the right ventricle, which causes delay in pulmonary valve closure (Leatham, 1975).

The intensity of the second heart sound can be highly suggestive of several cardiopulmonary disorders. The aortic component of the second sound will become louder in systemic hypertension and coarctation of the aorta, whereas emphysema and obesity will decrease the intensity of the aortic component of the second sound. The pulmonary component will be accentuated in pulmonary artery hypertension secondary to large left-to-right shunts such as in an atrial septal defect, ventricular septal defects, or patent ductus arteriosis. The intensity of the pulmonary component of the second heart sound will be decreased, or even absent, in severe pulmonic stenosis such as in tetralogy of Fallot.

To summarize, there are two normal sounds of the heart. The first sound coincides with the arterial pulse and is deeper and longer in duration than the second heart sound. The two sounds can also be distinguished by their rhythm; there is a longer pause between the second sound and the succeeding first sound than between the first and second sounds.

There is a type of abnormal heart sound called a *gallop sound* that warrants description. The term *gallop rhythm* describes an auscultatory phenomenon which resembles the cantor of a horse as the result of a tripling or even quadrupling of heart sounds. Gallop rhythms are diastolic events and are subdivided into atrial and ventricular gallop sounds, both of which are related to filling of the ventricles.

### Ventricular (S₃) Gallop

The ventricular gallop, or third heart sound, is frequently

one of the first signs indicating serious heart disease, although a normal physiologic third heart sound can be heard in some young individuals. The ventricular gallop occurs just after the second heart sound in the early part of diastole. It is generally believed the third heart sound is caused by oscillation of blood back and forth between the walls of the ventricles, initiated by the rushing of blood from the atria. It is heard most clearly when the patient is in the left lateral decubitus position during exhalation. Because this gallop rhythm is a low frequency sound, it is best heard with the bell of the stethoscope lightly applied to the skin over the point of maximum impulse (PMI). It is important to determine the PMI by palpation after the patient has assumed the left lateral decubitus position.

### Atrial (S₄) Gallop

The atrial gallop occurs during the presystolic filling phase related to atrial systole just prior to the first heart sound. Although this sound results from ventricular filling, it is more specifically related to atrial contraction. It is frequently heard in patients with coronary artery disease, hypertension, cardiopathies involving a delay in atrioventricular conduction, and also may be heard in some normal hearts. In fact, the atrial gallop may be one of the first clues from the physical examination to the presence of coronary artery disease. Like the ventricular gallop, the atrial gallop is most easily heard over the PMI with the bell chest piece and the patient in the left lateral position.

Differentiation between the $S_3$ and $S_4$ gallops requires careful listening to the temporal relationship of the first and second heart sounds. If the abnormal sound occurs just prior to the first heart sound, an atrial gallop is probably present. The abnormal sound more closely following the second heart sound is characteristic of a ventricular gallop.

### Valve Areas

The four valve areas are areas over the heart where the sounds of the valves have the most intensity. Although the order in which the valve areas are auscultated makes no difference, a routine should be adopted so that important findings are not omitted. The aortic valve area is located in the right second intercostal space just lateral to the sternum.

The tricuspid valve area is at the junction of the xiphoid process and the body of the sternum. The pulmonary valve area is in the second left intercostal space just lateral to the sternum and the mitral valve area is located in the fifth left intercostal space, 1 to 2 cm medial to the midclavicular line. As can be seen from *Figure 8-2*, the valve areas do not correspond to the anatomical location of the valves themselves.

One abnormal valve sound is an ejection click, which is a short, high-pitched sound heard at either the pulmonic area or the aortic area immediately after the first heart sound. A pulmonary ejection click suggests pulmonary valve stenosis, or, possibly, pulmonary hypertension. An aortic ejection click may occur with aortic valve stenosis, coarctation of the aorta or hypertension.

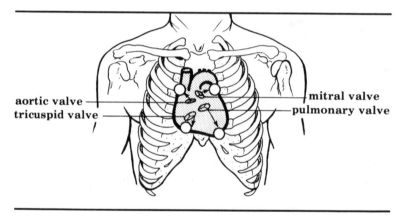

aortic valve
tricuspid valve
mitral valve
pulmonary valve

**Figure 8-2.** The anatomical location of the four heart valves. The areas where the sounds are heard best are shown as circles.

# Historical and Physical Findings in Specific Diseases

*Chapter Nine*

## HISTORICAL AND PHYSICAL FINDINGS
## IN SPECIFIC DISEASES

Since good clincial judgement depends on assimilating and synthesizing as many clues regarding the patient's state of well-being as possible, it is helpful to be aware of important findings from the patient history and physical examination concerning a particular disorder. The intent of this chapter is to present the hallmarks of the history and physical exam of some of the more common pulmonary problems seen in both the hospital and clinical settings. Since this discussion will be limited to the clinical aspects of various disorders, the reader should have a thorough understanding of the pathophysiology involved in each case.

### Asthma

**Definition:** Asthma is a chronic disease that has been difficult to define precisely in spite of increasing understanding of the pathophysiologic mechanisms involved. Asthma is a disease characterized by an increased responsiveness of the airways to various stimuli and manifested by widespread narrowing of the airways that changes in severity either spontaneously or as the result of therapy (American Thoracic Society, 1962). This definition of asthma purposefully omits any mention of specific etiologies or immunologic mechanisms because there are many factors which can precipitate an acute attack, and depending upon the type of asthma, the significance of immunologic mechanisms can be questionable. Rather, this definition describes a functional abnormality that is common to all asthmatics — hyper-reactivity of bronchial smooth muscle that is reversible.

**History:** In cases in which the patient can provide a detailed account of an acute attack, the history can be quite informative. The patient with extrinsic (allergic type) asthma will usually admit to a history of allergies and often specific allergens which have precipitated previous attacks. The extrinsic asthmatic will also admit to an onset of asthma in childhood or early adult life. A family history of multiple allergies is also common in these asthmatics. The intrinsic asthmatic is more difficult to detect because in his case there is usually no history of external allergens or family history of allergies. During the history, information concerning the duration, frequency, and severity of the attacks should be obtained. It is most important to ascertain the duration and course of the current disability in terms of the time of onset and the duration of the attacks and the effects of exposure to allergens, emotional stress, or unusual exertion. It is also necessary to determine whether a cough is present and, if so, the severity of the cough. In asthma, cough is initially nonproductive and increases in severity. Finally, it is imperative to determine the names, doses, and frequencies of administration of any medications the patient is taking. It is not unusual to uncover a history in which the patient increases dosages and self-administers medications on a more frequent basis in order to get relief.

There may be situations in which the patient is too dyspneic to provide a history. In such a case, a relative can often provide helpful information. And the initial evaluation will be much more productive if the clinician is aware of how long the patient has had the disease and knows something about the patient's current life situation.

The results of a physical examination of an asthmatic patient can vary considerably because the results depend upon the status of the patient at the time of the examination. Between attacks, the patient may be asymptomatic and appear entirely normal. During an attack, however, several characteristic signs of asthma will be noticeable.

**Inspection:** During a severe acute attack, the asthmatic patient is in obvious distress. The patient's mental status may be clouded to the point of confusion and even approaching coma, in which case carbon dioxide retention is suggested. By listening to the patient's speech pattern, one can get an idea of the degree of dyspnea the patient is experiencing. The patient who is able to say only three or four words before taking in a breath is experiencing greater dyspnea than the patient who can calmly relate an entire medical history without becoming short of breath. The skin of the asthmatic in acute distress is usually diaphoretic, pale, or cyanotic. Evidence of dehydration may also be present. Thoracic movement is slight due to the hyperinflated state of the lungs; this gives the patient a "barrel chest" appearance. Supraclavicular retractions and use of the accessory muscles of inspiration are commonly seen. Because of the severe shortness of breath, the patient's respiratory rate is often elevated to 30 to 40 breaths per minute, and the respiratory pattern typically shows expiration much longer in duration than inspiration.

**Palpation:** Palpation will confirm diminished chest wall movement in the acute asthmatic patient. The examiner will also note decreased vocal fremitus if hyperinflation is severe; otherwise, palpation is of minimal value in the physical examination of the patient with asthma.

**Percussion:** Percussion of the chest of an asthmatic usually elicits a hyperresonant note, but this depends upon the degree of hyperinflation present. The note resulting from percussion of an asthmatic may be resonant if the patient is not in an acute attack. During an acute episode, the hemidiaphragms can be noted to be depressed due to the hyperexpanded chest.

**Auscultation:** The nature of the breath sounds heard during a physical examination is influenced to a large extent by the severity of the disease at the time of the examination. During a mild attack of asthma, auscultation will reveal diminished breath sounds with wheezing on expiration. As the episode worsens, wheezing can be heard during both phases of respiration without the aid of a stethoscope. In a severe attack, breath sounds may be completely absent, which is an ominous sign of a total lack of ventilation. To reiterate, chest auscultation may also be normal between attacks.

**Chest Radiology:** Chest radiographs are not diagnostic of asthma. During an attack, the chest may appear normal or show signs of hyperinflation such as depressed hemidiaphragms and increased radiolucency. Occasionally, scattered densities may appear throughout the central and peripheral lung fields; these represent areas of atelectasis secondary to mucus plugs in the airways.

In summary, asthma is not as difficult to diagnose and treat as other pulmonary disorders. Many clinicians are, however, reluctant to tell the patient he or she has asthma simply because wheezing is present, and rightly so. The adage, "All that wheezes is not asthma" is very true, for there are many cardiopulmonary disorders that can cause wheezing. If the patient responds favorably to asthma drugs, an asthmatic component can be said to exist. The majority of asthma cases can be correctly diagnosed and treated with the help of a good history and physical examination.

## Emphysema

**Definition:** Pulmonary emphysema is generally defined as an anatomical alteration of the lung characterized by an abnormal enlargement of the airspaces distal to the terminal, nonrespiratory bronchiole accompanied by destructive changes of the alveolar walls. This definition describes emphysema in its pure form. In practical terms, emphysema often coexists with chronic bronchitis and it can be difficult to distinguish these two different pathological entities. Knowledge of the following characteristic signs of emphysema will help the clinician to determine whether emphysema is present:

1. Expiratory flow obstruction not significantly improved with bronchodilator administration.

2. Elevated total lung capacity and residual volume determinations.

3. Elastic recoil is low and lung compliance is high.

4. The diffusing capacity for carbon monoxide is decreased.

**History:** The medical history of the patient, though not diagnostic, is useful in determining whether emphysema is present. Inquiry should be made into the patient's past medical history because repeated respiratory infections in childhood may lead to chronic airway obstruction in later life. The patient should also be questioned in detail about the presence of a cough during the course of the disease. The majority of patients with emphysema will have a chronic cough and expectoration at some time during the disease process, and many patients will reveal that a productive cough was one of the first symptoms.

Another important aspect of the clinical picture of the patient with emphysema is a history of inappropriate dyspnea on exertion. This dyspnea often worsens when the

150

patient contracts what seems to be a severe chest cold that lingers on for weeks or months. One should ascertain the conditions under which the patient becomes dyspneic and whether this dyspnea has worsened.

Because of the direct relationship between tobacco abuse and the incidence of emphysema, a detailed smoking history of the patient is extremely helpful. Whether cigarette smoking is a cause of emphysema is not exactly known; however, most observers believe that cigarette smoking is a major cause of chronic bronchitis, which is commonly a precursor of centrilobular emphysema.

As chronic airway obstruction advances without treatment, the clincial features diverge into a group of symptoms, the two extremes of which can be easily identified. One extreme is the type A or "pink puffer," who suffers from emphysema, and the other extreme, type B or "blue bloater," has chronic bronchitis. These clear-cut extremes become apparent only in latter stages of airway obstruction.

The clinical manifestations of pulmonary emphysema vary from patient to patient. Some pulmonary emphysema sufferers are asymptomatic or have no abnormal physical signs even though emphysema is found at autopsy, while symptomatic patients have clinical alterations which are found in a number of diseases. The following clinical features depict the patient with pure, uncomplicated emphysema.

**Inspection:** One of the first clinical findings noted in the patient with emphysema is dyspnea. This is manifested by tachypnea with shallow respirations, a prolonged expiratory phase, and use of the accessory muscles. The emphysematous patient is often cachetic with a barrel-shaped chest. Inspection of the chest discloses widened intercostal spaces and a wider-than-normal costal angle. It is not unusual for this patient to prefer to sit leaning forward in order to gain some mechanical advantage for the accessory muscles. This posture in combination with the barrel-chest gives the impression of accentuated thoracic kyphosis. Also, the patient often uses "pursed-lip" breathing to prevent premature airway closure during expiration. Digital clubbing and cyanosis are both unusual in the type A patient. The latter is uncommon because these patients are able to maintain their arterial oxygen saturation ($SaO_2$) by hyperventilating and also keep the arterial carbon dioxide tension ($PaCO_2$) within normal limits until the final stages of the disease; hence the name "pink puffer." If cyanosis is present, a bronchial carcinoma or bronchiectasis should be suspected.

**Palpation:** Tactile fremitus is decreased in patients with chronic emphysema because of the excessive amount of air between the larynx and the chest wall. Likewise, the point of maximal impulse will be diminished because of an increased retrosternal airspace which will minimize the cardiac vibrations reaching the chest wall. The hyperinflation of the lungs will also cause a shift of the heart to a more vertical position resulting in a medial shift in the PMI.

Decreased lateral movement of the chest wall can be detected with chest palpation. Because of the abnormal chest wall configuration and accessory muscle use, the thorax tends to move up and down rather than laterally.

**Percussion:** The percussion note heard most commonly over the chest of the patient with severe emphysema is hyperresonant. This finding, too, is secondary to lung hyperinflation. At times the hyperinflation is so severe that areas of the chest which are normally dull to percussion, such as over the heart or liver, will be hyperresonant. This is one of the most dramatic findings on percussion of the chest.

When percussing the posterior thorax for diaphragmatic movement, one will often find a decrease in diaphragmatic excursion. In fact, in severe emphysema, diaphragmatic movement may not be detected at all because the hemidiaphragms are pushed down in a horizontal position and do not move on inspiration.

**Auscultation:** Listening to the chest of the patient with uncomplicated emphysema reveals breath sounds which are rather nonspecific. Typically, the breath sounds are diminished, there are no adventitious sounds, and the expiratory phase is considerably longer than the inspiratory phase of respiration; however, these features are characteristic of any pathology involving an increased thoracic gas volume and airway obstruction. The voice sounds are also decreased, but they are of little help in the physical diagnosis of emphysema. Like the lung sounds, the heart sounds are also low in intensity.

**Chest radiology:** The chest radiograph of the emphysema patient may be deceptively normal until advanced disease is present, at which time an increased radiolucency throughout both lung fields will be revealed (assuming proper exposure). This is accompanied by a loss of pulmonary vascular markings and low, flattened diaphragms often with *interdigitation* (a scalloped appearance). The cardiac shadow is small and elongated, particularly on deep inspiration. In a lateral view, an increased retrosternal airspace can often be appreciated. These radiographic characteristics are classic features of advanced emphysema.

## Chronic Bronchitis

**Definition:** Chronic bronchitis is a disease that has been defined in clinical terms for a long time. Chronic bronchitis is a clinical disorder characterized by excessive mucus secretion in the bronchial tree which is manifested by chronic or recurrent productive cough. These manifestations should be present on most days for a minimum of three months in the year and for not less than two successive years (American Thoracic Society, 1962). Since many diseases, such as tuberculosis, lung abscess, and bronchiectasis, have similar manifestations, a diagnosis of chronic bronchitis should not be made without having first excluded these other disorders as possible causes of the symptoms.

Pathologically, chronic bronchitis is characterized by hypertrophy and hyperplasia of the mucous glands. This results in an increase in the ratio of the bronchial gland thickness to the bronchial wall thickness. If pathologic findings were used to define chronic bronchitis, the diagnosis would be relatively easy; however, because these findings cannot be conveniently obtained, clinicians must rely on the results of pulmonary function tests to recognize chronic bronchitis. The patient with pure chronic bronchitis should demonstrate the following:

1. Expiratory and inspiratory flow obstruction which is not significantly improved with bronchodilator administration.

2. Normal lung volumes with only slight elevation of the RV/TLC ratio.

3. Normal lung compliance.

4. Normal diffusing capacity for carbon monoxide.

5. Hypoxemia without hypercapnea.

**History:** Many of the patients with chronic bronchitis are so accustomed to the symptoms of cough and dyspnea that they are often unaware of the presence of these symptoms. In fact, some patients will even deny any symptoms. It is therefore helpful to have the spouse present during the interview.

Typically, upon careful questioning, the patient will admit to a progressive cough with expectoration. This cough usually begins as a "smoker's cough," only present in the morning, and gradually worsens over a period of months. Some patients have a history of frequent upper respiratory infections during which time the cough becomes more severe and sputum production increases.

The most important factor associated with the etiology of chronic bronchitis is airway irritation from cigarette smoking. The severity of chronic bronchitis is also directly related to the number of cigarettes smoked. In persons with chronic bronchitis who give up smoking, the cough diminishes, and they will usually admit to an improvement in exercise tolerance. If smoking is not stopped until latter stages of the disease, the benefits are almost undetectable.

Physical findings vary considerably depending upon whether the patient is experiencing an exacerbation of a respiratory infection. The clinical picture of the patient with chronic bronchitis depicts a person with dyspnea and a chronic cough with expectoration. As the disease progresses, clinical features of the type B or "blue bloater" syndrome become apparent.

**Inspection:** Patients with pure chronic bronchitis are typically normal to obese in body stature. During an exacerbation of a respiratory infection, cyanosis is often present as well as dependent edema and jugular venous distension secondary to right ventricular failure; hence the description of "blue bloater". These patients can also demonstrate exertional dyspnea which is usually episodic rather than progressive in character. If the shortness of breath is severe, accessory muscle use will be obvious. Contrary to the type A individual, a barrel-chest is not common in the person with pure chronic bronchitis.

154

**Palpation:** Thoracic palpation is usually unremarkable in the patient with pure chronic bronchitis unless the disease is complicated by pneumonia. When this is the case, one would expect vocal fremitus to be increased. Palpation of the liver and the extremities might yield further evidence of right heart failure such as an enlarged, sometimes pulsating liver and pitting edema.

**Percussion:** In patients with uncomplicated chronic bronchitis, a normal, resonant percussion note is the rule. If pneumonia is also present, the percussion note will be dull; if emphysema exists concommitantly, not only will a hyper-resonant note be present, but diaphragmatic excursion will be reduced. Abdominal percussion will confirm an enlarged liver evidenced by an increased area of dullness over the right upper quadrant.

**Auscultation:** As with other parts of the physical examination, the results of chest auscultation are dependent upon the severity of the bronchitis and the presence of any other disease processes. In uncomplicated chronic bronchitis, breath sounds are essentially normal; however, there is generally a prolonged expiratory time. Since many patients with chronic bronchitis have abundant secretions, low-pitched wheezes are commonly heard.

Depending upon body stature and the degree of hyperinflation present, the heart sounds in the patient with chronic bronchitis can be either normal or diminished in intensity. In patients who have significant pulmonary hyperinflation, the heart sounds will be diminished in intensity. Because right ventricular hypertrophy is common in these patients, one can often hear an accentuated pulmonary closure sound and a right ventricular $S_3$ gallop.

**Chest Radiology:** Patients with chronic bronchitis uncomplicated by emphysema often have normal chest radiographs. The lung fields are normal in size with a slight increase in vascular markings. As pulmonary hypertension develops late in the course of the disease, the pulmonary artery shadows become more prominent and the cardiac silhouette enlarges. Otherwise, the chest radiograph is not much help in the diagnosis of chronic bronchitis.

## Pneumonia

**Definition:** The term *pneumonia* indicates an inflammatory response, generally acute, of the lungs. This inflammation is usually the result of a bacterial, viral, fungal, mycobacterial, or chemical infection of the lungs. Because of the structure of the lungs, infectious agents can enter the lungs via two routes: inhalation into the airways, which is the most common route, and by the blood in the pulmonary and bronchial arterial circulations.

Pneumonia begins with inflammation of the bronchioles resulting in alveolar filling with pus, red blood cells, plasma, and the infecting organisms. This produces an airless consolidation of lung tissue in the affected area. The history and physical findings of pneumonia depend upon the type of pneumonia, its severity, and the time during the course of the disease that the examination is performed. For example, patients with pneumococcal pneumonia initially spike a temperature and often complain of pleuritic pain over the affected area. The cough is initially dry, but soon becomes productive of purulent sputum. On the other hand, patients with viral pneumonia exhibit symptoms different from those of a bacterial pneumonia. There is seldom pleuritic pain, sputum is often mucoid, and the white blood cell count is normal in the early stages of the disease.

**History:** Because the presenting symptoms vary with the type of pneumonia, the history will differ from patient to patient. Approximately half the patients with bacterial pneumonia complain of an upper respiratory infection followed by evidence of lower respiratory tract involvement. Classic manifestations of bacterial pneumonia include fever, cough, and chest pain. The fever generally ranges from 100° to 106°F. and is frequently accompanied by teeth-chattering chills. The cough is productive in the majority of patients and the sputum may have the classic rusty appearance or may be purulent. As was previously mentioned, the chest pain is usually pleuritic, increasing in intensity during a deep inspiration or cough.

Most patients with viral pneumonia have an underlying cardiopulmonary disease or are pregnant. Initial symptoms are similar to those associated with influenza. Within 24 to 36 hours, however, the patient is aware of increasing shortness of breath and a slightly productive cough. Otherwise, there may be little in the way of respiratory symptoms. There are, though, exceptions to this clinical history. If the underlying disease is severe, the patient may demonstrate more respiratory symptoms other than dyspnea and a productive cough. Tachypnea as well as accessory muscle use may also be evident. Also, these symptoms may not take as long as 24 to 36 hours to become evident. All patients with viral pneumonia do not present identical histories.

**Inspection:** Physical examination of the patient with pneumonia often reveals a diaphoretic, acutely ill individual. The patient usually exhibits tachypnea accompanied by shallow respirations. This results in limited chest movement, particularly on the affected side. The presence of pleuritic pain also contributes to decreased inspiratory movement. In more severe cases, nasal flaring and the use of the accessory muscles can be noted. Cyanosis is uncommon in pneumonia except in the most severe cases.

**Palpation:** Thoracic palpation can contribute to the diagnosis of pneumonia. If there is a significant consolidation of lung tissue, one should expect to find decreased chest movement on the affected side. When palpating for tracheal deviation, the examiner will generally find the trachea midline unless the consolidation is massive. If this is the case, the trachea as well as the apex heart beat will be shifted *away* from the affected side.

In patients whose pneumonia has resulted in consolidation, vocal fremitus will be increased. In some patients, though, the pneumonic process will result in a secondary pleural effusion in which vocal fremitus will be decreased. Also, if airways between the larynx and the affected area of lung are filled with secretions, this will decrease vocal fremitus by blocking the transmission of vibrations from the larynx. Therefore, if pneumonia is suspected and fremitus is decreased, instruct the patient to cough and test for vocal fremitus again. Vocal fremitus is only helpful in diagnosing pneumonia when it is increased, and is of minimal value when it is normal or decreased.

**Percussion:** Depending upon the stage of the pneumonia at the time of the examination, the percussion note may be dull, flat, or resonant. When the disease process is moderately advanced, the affected area of the lung will be filled with fluid and cellular material, resulting in a dull percussion

157

note. As this process worsens, the affected area will become airless and the percussion note will approach very dull or flat in character. In cases where the pneumonia is diffuse, there may be enough aerated areas to result in a resonant note. For the most part, pneumonia will result in a dull percussion note.

**Auscultation:** The results of auscultating the chest of the patient with pneumonia also depend upon the severity and the course of the disease when the examination is performed. In the early stages of pneumonia, breath sounds are essentially normal. As the pneumonia worsens, the breath sounds become hollow or tubular in quality. This results from the consolidated lung tissue filtering the lower frequency sounds before they reach the chest wall, thereby allowing only the higher-pitched sounds to reach the chestpiece. As fluid from the pneumonia begins to fill the terminal airways, one can hear late inspiratory crackles, particularly at the lung bases. In advanced pneumonia, fluid and mucus enter the large airways which decreases the lumen of the airways and results in low-pitched wheezes.

Voice sounds will be abnormal in patients whose areas of pneumonia have become completely consolidated. Since consolidated lung tissue transmits spoken and whispered sounds more clearly, bronchophony as well as whispered pectoriloquy will be present over the area of consolidation. If there is doubt whether a pleural effusion is also present, the examiner should test for egophony.

**Chest Radiology:** The radiographic signs of pneumonia may vary considerably with the specific etiology; however, there are general signs that are frequently seen. A consolidation will appear as an area of increased radiodensity which may involve one or more segments, a lobe, or one or both lungs. If the pneumonia is contained within a single segment or lobe, it will have sharp borders delineating the area of involvement. If the pneumonic process involves several segments, but not an entire lobe, it will appear as a poorly outlined, patchy opacity. If the pneumonia involves the lung parenchyma, but the airways are patent and not filled with secretions, air bronchograms can often be visualized.

## Pulmonary Fibrosis

**Definition:** Fibrosis is the formation of connective (scar) tissue in the lung or pleura as the result of the healing process in response to an inflammatory process. Pulmonary fibrosis can be localized, such as that which may follow necrotizing pneumonia, or it can be a widespread disease involving both lungs.

The causes of widespread lung injury resulting in diffuse pulmonary fibrosis usually fall into the categories listed in Table 9-1. Fibrotic changes can occur in varying degrees in each of these categories. Because of this, the clinical manifestations are proportional to the pattern of scar tissue distribution.

**Table 9-1. Causes of diffuse fibrosis.**

1. extrinsic allergic alveolitis
2. sarcoidosis
3. inorganic dust pneumoconiosis
4. connective tissue diseases
5. irradiation
6. pulmonary infections
7. oxygen toxicity
8. idiopathy

The interstitial changes associated with diffuse pulmonary fibrosis are characteristic of a restrictive lesion. A restrictive lesion is manifested by a decreased vital capacity and total lung capacity but a normal FEV/FVC ratio. A reduction in the diffusing capacity of carbon monoxide is probably the earliest change in pulmonary function. The arterial oxygen tension may be normal early in the disease process; however, as blood continues to be shunted through the perfused but underventilated lung, chronic hypoxemia will develop. This hypoxemia will result in pulmonary artery vasoconstriction which contributes to the elevated pulmonary artery pressure.

**History:** Dyspnea is the primary symptom in patients with advanced pulmonary fibrosis. Initially, patients are only dyspneic on exertion but later they are also dyspneic at rest. The clinician should inquire about the possibility of any disease-inducing occupational exposure to noxious fumes, gases or other irritating substances, or repeated respiratory infections which might lead to fibrotic lung changes. The physical examination may be significant or perfectly normal, depending upon the severity of pulmonary fibrosis and the presence of any concomitant illness. For this reason a lung biopsy is used in most instances to make the diagnosis.

**Inspection:** Patients with moderate to advanced pulmonary fibrosis are quite often short of breath. In fact, a complaint of dyspnea often precedes any other signs of pulmonary embarrassment. The relationship between the degree of dyspnea and the amount of exertion is an indication of the severity of the disease; if the patient is short of breath during minimal exertion, the fibrosis may be advanced. Along with the shortness of breath, patients will demonstrate marked tachypnea with shallow respirations. Inspection will reveal limited chest expansion, particularly in patients with an advanced case of pulmonary fibrosis. Cyanosis is at first present only during exercise but later may occur while the patient is at rest. If there is a secondary infection associated with the disease, a productive cough with purulent sputum will be present. Otherwise, cough is not a common symptom. Digital clubbing is common but not always seen.

**Palpation:** Palpating the chest wall will confirm the decreased thoracic expansion noted during inspection. By systematically testing vocal fremitus, the examiner can approximate the distribution of the fibrosis in each lung. Since solid, fibrotic lung tissue transmits voice vibrations better than normal lung parenchyma, fremitus will be increased over the areas of involvement. Normally, the trachea is midline; however, if the fibrosis is significantly greater in one lung than the other, the trachea will tend to deviate *toward* the more affected side.

**Percussion:** Determination of diaphragmatic excursion will reveal limited movement of both hemidiaphragms. If the fibrosis is more severe on one side, one will expect less diaphragmatic movement on that side. Percussion over the lung fields produces a dull note. In more severe cases, the percussion note will be very dull or even flat. If compensatory emphysema is present in an unaffected lung, expect the note to be hyperresonant on that side (Druger, 1973).

**Auscultation:** Breath sounds in the patient with diffuse pulmonary fibrosis are usually diminished in intensity. In regard to adventitious sounds, diffuse crackles are often heard at the lung bases, particularly during a deep inspiration. These crackles are believed to be the result of the extension of fibrotic tissue. Low-pitched wheezes are not common unless an infection is also present.

Abnormal voice sounds are usually present over areas of fibrotic lung tissue. Both whispered pectoriloquy and bronchophony will be increased and, as the lung tissue becomes more dense, these voice sounds will become louder.

**Chest Radiology:** The chest roentgenogram may be normal in the early stages of the disease, in spite of dyspnea. As the fibrosis worsens, the lung fields on the radiograph show a diffuse, "ground glass" appearance. Occasionally one can observe a streaky pattern of shadows, especially at the lung bases.

## Atelectasis

**Definition:** The word *atelectasis* comes from the Greek derivation *ateles* (imperfect) and *ektasis* (expansion). It is generally used to describe partial or complete collapse of lung tissue and can involve an area as small as a single lung unit or as much as both lungs. It is one of the most common complications and occurs in patients with or without pulmonary disease.

There are two types of atelectasis, which are distinguished by their causes: compression atelectasis and obstructive atelectasis. Compression atelectasis can develop in an entire lung or part of a lung as a result of pressure applied from an extrapulmonary source such as a pleural effusion, a pneumothorax or severe cardiomegaly. Obstructive atelectasis develops as a result of an occlusion of a bronchus or a bronchiole, and the air in the alveoli distal to the obstruction gets absorbed into the bloodstream. The involved alveoli begin to shrink to a critical volume below which they eventually collapse. In obstructive atelectasis, the lung does not pull away from the chest wall; it merely becomes smaller. Causes of obstructive atelectasis include retained secretions, endobronchial tumor or foreign body aspiration.

Atelectasis is also a common post-operative complication following thoracic and upper abdominal surgery. Some of the conditions which predispose a patient to this common problem include pain, sedation, immobility, splinting of the diaphragm, and surgical dressings, all of which contribute to a reduction in ventilation. When an infection or fluid overload is superimposed on these post-operative conditions, pulmonary atelectasis is virtually inevitable.

**History:** Information contained in the history provided by the patient will depend upon the cause of the atelectasis. In compressive atelectasis, because the primary disease may mask the pulmonary changes, the patient may complain of pain, dyspnea, or cough long before the signs of atelectasis are apparent. If the atelectasis is caused by an endobronchial tumor, the symptoms develop quite slowly. When atelectasis is caused by an obstruction such as secretions or a foreign body, symptoms including cough, dyspnea, and fever develop rapidly.

Certain historical information should help the clinician to discover the cause of the atelectasis. For example, if atelectasis is seen on a post-operative chest radiograph, one should consider the possible causes of post-operative atelectasis mentioned above. If atelectasis is present in a middle-aged individual with a history of cigarette smoking, one should be suspicious of a carcinoma obstructing a bronchus.

The results of the physical examination will vary depending upon the severity of atelectasis. If the atelectasis only involves a small area of the lung, the physical signs may be completely normal. If a lobar or mainstem bronchus is occluded, however, the signs and symptoms will be dramatic.

**Inspection:** When a mainstem bronchus is obstructed, the patient appears anxious and distressed. The respiratory rate is increased and cyanosis is often present due to blood flowing through non-ventilated areas of the lung. The hemithorax on the affected side appears smaller than the hemithorax on the unaffected side, and shows a narrowing of the intercostal spaces. Chest movement on the involved side will be diminished while the uninvolved side appears hyperexpanded, with the ribs assuming a more horizontal position. Observation of the PMI reveals a shift toward the affected side.

**Palpation:** Thoracic palpation is helpful in confirming the findings revealed during inspection. The chest wall on the side of the atelectasis can be felt to move less than the unaffected side. If the atelectasis is considerable, the trachea will be shifted *toward* the atelectatic side. The PMI will be shifted to the left and slightly upward if the left lung is involved and toward the midline with right-sided atelectasis. Since the voice vibrations are blocked as they enter the atelectatic area, tactile fremitus will be significantly reduced or absent.

**Percussion:** Because of the airless lung tissue under the chest wall, percussion yields a dull note over atelectatic areas. In contrast, the percussion note over an unaffected, aerated lung will be hyperresonant because of compensatory emphysema (Kampmeier, 1970). This is a term used to describe the overinflation that occurs when a lung or part of a lung responds to fill a space previously occupied by an aerated lung tissue. Testing for diaphragmatic excursion can help determine the extent of the atelectasis. If the involved area is small, diaphragmatic excursion may be equal on both sides. If the atelectasis is significant, the examiner should expect decreased movement on the affected side with possible elevation of that hemidiaphragm.

Another technique useful in determining the severity of the atelectasis involves locating the area of cardiac dullness by percussion. If the right lung is completely atelectatic, the heart may be shifted far enough to the right that the borders of cardiac dullness cannot be determined. The right heart border will be confluent with the consolidated lung tissue and the left heart border will be under the sternum.

**Auscultation:** Breath sounds will usually be diminished or absent over atelectatic areas. Rarely, such as when a bronchus is partially obstructed and air can enter and leave the terminal airways, the breath sounds assume a tubular quality. Adventitious lung sounds are not generally heard over areas of atelectasis. In some post-operative patients, however, basal crackles may be present, but they should gradually diminish after several deep inspirations. Testing for this diminishing pattern of crackles will help the examiner rule out other pathological causes of crackles such as congestive heart failure and pneumonia. Voice sounds are usually decreased in intensity because vocal vibrations are prevented from reaching the chest wall.

**Chest Radiology:** Even though radiographic examination is very helpful in diagnosing atelectasis, the radiograph may be normal when small areas of the lung are involved. When atelectasis is significant, there will be both direct and indirect signs of its presence on a chest radiograph. Direct signs include increased radiodensity and volume loss in an entire lung or lobe. Indirect signs of atelectasis include elevation of a hemidiaphragm, crowded intercostal spaces, displaced fissures, and a mediastinal shift toward the affected side. In patients who have undergone upper abdominal or thoracic surgery, platelike atelectasis is frequently seen. This term is used to describe horizontal shadows of increased density in lower lobes which were compressed during surgery and have not fully re-expanded.

## Pleural Effusion

**Definition:** In the normal individual, the visceral and parietal pleurae are lubricated by a small amount of thin fluid which facilitates the movement of the lungs within the thorax. A pleural effusion exists when there is an abnormal accumulation of fluid in the pleural space. Pleural effusion is a sign of pre-existing disease and not a disease entity in itself.

A pleural effusion may result from a number of different conditions which cause increased formation of fluid in the intrapleural space, decreased absorption of pleural fluid, or a combination of these two. In order to help determine the etiology, pleural effusions are classified as transudates or exudates, depending upon their mechanism of formation and chemical composition. A transudate is usually the result of an imbalance between the transcapillary pressure and plasma oncotic pressure. An exudate results from increased capillary permeability due to inflammation or carcinoma. Typically, transudates are clear or slightly yellow fluids with a low protein content, low specific gravity, and very few cellular components. In contrast, exudates are dark yellow or cloudy fluids with higher protein contents and higher specific gravity. Exudates also contain many white blood cells. Transudates often occur bilaterally compared to exudates, which are usually unilateral. Specific causes of pleural transudates and exudates are listed in Table 9-2.

**Table 9-2. Causes of pleural effusion.**

| Transudates | Exudates |
| --- | --- |
| congestive heart failure | infectious diseases (tuberculosis, bacterial pneumonia) |
| cirrhosis of the liver | neoplasms |
| renal failure | surgery and/or trauma |
| vascular obstruction | post myocardial infarction |
| | acute pancreatitis |

Pleural effusions are also described on the basis of their composition. If the effusion consists primarily of a watery fluid, the term *hydrothorax* is used to describe the effusion. If the fluid is infected and there is pus in the pleural space, the terms *empyema* or *pyothorax* are used. If the pleural fluid is bloody, as may occur after trauma, the term *hemothorax* is used to describe the effusion. If there is a leakage of chyle into the pleural space from obstruction or trauma to the thoracic duct, a *chylothorax* is present. The exact content of the fluid, however, cannot be determined without the aid of a diagnostic pleural tap or *thoracentesis*.

**History:** Since a pleural effusion is often the result of a pre-existing disease, the patient history will more closely correlate with the primary condition. If the underlying problem is congestive heart failure, for example, the orthopnea and the paroxysmal nocturnal dyspnea of which the patient complains and the noticeable jugular venous distension are all secondary to the heart failure and not to the effusion. In a few patients, however, the signs and symptoms associated with the pleural effusion will be the only ones present. The severity of these symptoms will vary with both the amount of fluid present and the rapidity with which the fluid has developed. When the amount of fluid is less than 100 ml, it is virtually undetectable in the adult. A chest radiograph can detect as little as 300 ml of fluid. The results of a physical examination will be unrevealing unless there is at least 500 ml of fluid present (Crofton, 1975).

**Inspection:** Upon inspection of the patient with a pleural effusion, one will notice restricted chest excursion on the affected side. This is due to the fluid compressing the lung tissue and inhibiting expansion. In the patient with a massive effusion, the lower intercostal spaces on the affected side can actually bulge outward. The respiratory rate is generally increased. Cyanosis is not usually present unless a massive, bilateral pleural effusion exists.

**Palpation:** In pleural effusions of moderate size (1,000 ml), thoracic palpation confirms the limited chest movement on the involved side noticed during inspection. Tracheal palpation reveals a deviation away from the affected side of the thorax. Vocal fremitus is either diminished or absent, particularly along the lateral chest wall and posteriorly at the lung bases. In a massive effusion, the area of absent fremitus may extend up to the apex of the lung on the involved side when the patient is in the upright position. In a right-sided effusion, the PMI will be shifted to the left and in a left-sided effusion, the PMI may not be felt at all because it is under the sternum.

**Percussion:** Percussion directly over a pleural effusion will yield a dull percussion note; however, percussion *above* the level of the effusion in an erect individual often yields a hyperresonant note. This is due to overexpansion of alveoli compensating for the compressed alveoli under the effusion. To help quantitate the pleural effusion, it is important to determine the upper level of the effusion posteriorly by percussing from the apex downward until a dull percussion note is heard. (This same procedure is performed when a thoracentesis is required.) Recognition of this dull note may be slightly difficult in a right-sided effusion because the dullness of the effusion merges with the liver dullness. In a left-sided effusion, the percussion note may abruptly change from dull to tympanic as one percusses downward and reaches the stomach bubble. Also, the amount of shift in the area of cardiac dullness is proportional to the severity of the effusion — the greater the shift, the more fluid is probably present.

**Auscultation:** Lung and voice sounds are quite variable and are dependent upon the amount of fluid present. Breath sounds are diminished or absent because they are blocked before they reach the stethoscope chestpiece. If the effusion is small and the pleural surfaces are roughened and rub together, a pleural friction rub may be heard, particularly in the lung bases. This friction rub will disappear as the effusion increases in volume. There are no other adventitious sounds unique to a pleural effusion.

When auscultating over the area of a pleural effusion, the voice sounds will be attenuated. To help differentiate between a consolidation and an effusion, egophony will be present just above the level of the effusion.

**Chest Radiology:** Because of the charcteristic shadow the pleural effusion produces, the chest radiograph is the definitive diagnostic procedure for a pleural effusion. It usually appears as a dense, homogenous opacity occupying the lower part of the chest in an upright radiograph. (Remember, fluid moves to the gravity dependent areas of the chest.) The costophrenic angle on the involved hemithorax will be obliterated and the upper border of the fluid will have a concave downward curve with the highest level in the axillary area. In the aerated lung immediately above the effusion, one will readily notice an air-fluid level. To determine if the effusion is comprised of free, moving fluid or if it is loculated, a lateral decubitus radiograph is recommended. If the fluid is free to move, it will layer out along the lateral chest wall. A loculated effusion will usually remain within its cavity, such as in an interlobar fissure, or between the diaphragm and the inferior pulmonary surface (subpulmonic effusion).

## Pneumothorax

**Definition:** Pneumothorax, the presence of air in the pleural space, is a common clinical condition. It can be classified into three general types, open, closed, or tension pneumothorax, depending upon the mechanism of its formation.

In an *open pneumothorax,* there is either a direct communication between the pleural space and the atmosphere (external) or between the pleural space and the lung (internal). In both cases, the pressure of the air in the pleural space will be atmospheric. The most common cause is a chest wall injury, such as a stab wound, resulting in an external communication. Common causes of an internal communication include a spontaneous rupture of a pulmonary bleb and a bronchopleural fistula.

A *closed pneumothorax* refers to air in the pleural space that is not in communication with the air in the lungs or the atmosphere. This type of pneumothorax may occur when air

167

has leaked into the pleural space from the lung and the site of the leak has sealed. Examples of this include the rupture of a subpleural bleb or when air is accidentally introduced into the pleural space.

A *tension pneumothorax* refers to air that enters the pleural space from the lung only in inspiration, and on expiraton the air leak is sealed by a one-way valve mechanism that prevents its exit. Therefore, intrapleural pressure increases with each breath, eventually exceeding atmospheric pressure. This increasing pressure will result in collapse of the lung on the side of the pneumothorax, and compression of the great vessels resulting in a drop in cardiac output. A tension pneumothorax is considered a medical emergency and can lead to death if intervention is not immediate.

**History:** The clinical history and physical findings in pneumothorax depend upon the amount of air in the intrapleural space and the extent of lung collapse. In the majority of patients, the symptoms are mild, but in some patients, symptoms are quite severe. *Pain* is, by far, the most common symptom. It is usually acute in onset, very sharp, and aggravated by respiration. This pain is usually localized to the low lateral portion of the chest, although it may radiate to almost any location. Dyspnea is the other symptom of which patients will frequently complain; it is often severe and the patient is in obvious respiratory distress. The patient is unable to inspire deeply, which results in increased respiratory effort in order to fill the lungs completely. If the pneumothorax is minimal, the physical examination may be within normal limits; however, if the pneumothorax involves at least one-third of a lung, the physical findings are characteristic (Myerson, 1948).

**Inspection:** The clinical picture of the patient with a spontaneous pneumothorax typically reveals a young, otherwise healthy male complaining of dyspnea and chest pain. Also, the respiratory rate will usually be increased. The chest motion on the affected side is diminished, and in some cases, one can notice a bulging of the intercostal spaces on that same side. When the respiratory distress is significant, the accessory muscles will often be utilized. Cyanosis is usually not present unless the pneumothorax is under tension. If the pneumothorax is under tension, cyanosis may appear rapidly.

**Palpation:** Upon palpation, one will find the trachea deviated away from the side of the pneumothorax, especially when a tension pneumothorax is present. The PMI will also be shifted to the opposite side of the pneumothorax. Thoracic palpation also confirms decreased chest excursion on the affected side when compared to the unaffected side. In a moderate to large pneumothorax, tactile fremitus will be diminished or totally absent.

**Percussion:** The percussion note heard over an open and closed pneumothorax will be hyperresonant. If a tension pneumothorax is present, the percussion note will be tympanic. While percussing the chest, the clinician will notice that the area of cardiac dullness will be obliterated if the air is in the left pleural space.

**Auscultation:** The breath sounds in a patient with a pneumothorax are considerably diminished or even absent over the affected hemithorax. Because of the excessive amount of air in the pleural space, voice sounds will also be decreased. It may be difficult to distinguish between a pneumothorax and a large bulla in some patients, particularly in older patients in whom the onset of the pneumothorax is more gradual. The metallic coin test may provide the differentiation. In this test, the examiner holds a coin firmly against the anterior chest wall. When this coin is tapped with another while listening to the posterior chest with the stethoscope, a unique metallic ringing sound is heard over the areas of a pneumothorax and will not be heard over a bulla.

**Chest Radiology:** In the chest radiograph lies definitive diagnosis of pneumothorax. It is characterized by the clearly defined lung edge separated from the skeletal wall by a radiopaque zone which is devoid of pulmonary vascular markings. If the pneumothorax is small, it may be overlooked unless an expiratory radiograph is taken. With this technique, the size of the pneumothorax is exaggerated in comparison to the size of the lung, thereby making it more easily observable. A tension pneumothorax or a large open pneumothorax will result in a mediastinal shift *away* from the affected side.

Table 9-3 summarizes the physical findings associated with the disorders in this chapter.

**Table 9-3. Summary of physical findings in specific disorders.**

| | Asthma | Emphysema | Chronic Bronchitis | Pneumonia (R. lung) | Pulmonary Fibrosis | Atelectasis (R. lung) | Effusion (R. side) | Pneumothorax (R. lung) |
|---|---|---|---|---|---|---|---|---|
| Chest excursion | ↓R & L | ↓R & L | WNL | ↓R | ↓R & L | ↓R | ↓R | ↓R |
| Tracheal position | WNL | WNL | WNL | WNL; if massive→ L | WNL; if greater on R, →R | shift to R | shift to left | shift to left |
| Vocal fremitus | ↓R & L | ↓R & L | WNL | ↑R | ↑over affected area | ↓R | ↓ or absent | ↓ or absent |
| Percussion | hyper-resonant | hyper-resonant | resonant | dull | dull | dull | dull | hyper-resonant |
| Breath sounds | ↓R & L | ↓R& L | WNL | ↓R | ↓over affected area | ↓ or absent on right | ↓ or absent on right | ↓ or absent on right |
| Adventitious sounds | high-pitched wheezes | — | low-pitched wheezes | late inspiratory crackles Bronchophony Whispered pectoriloquy | crackles at bases | — | -friction rub -egophony just above fluid level | — |

# Bibliography

# BIBLIOGRAPHY

American Thoracic Society. "Chronic bronchitis, asthma, and pulmonary emphysema: A statement by the Committee on Diagnostic Standards for Nontuberculous Respiratory Diseases." *American Review of Respiratory Disease* 82 (1962): 762-68.

Barbee, R.A., S. Feldman, and L.W. Chosy. "The quantitative evaluation of student performance in the medical interview." *Journal of Medical Education* 42 (March 1967): 238-43.

Bates, B. *A Guide to Physical Examination.* Philadelphia: J.B. Lippincott, 1974.

Beard, R., E. Morris, and S. Clayton. "pH of foetal capillary blood as an indicator of the condition of the foetus." *J. Obstet Gynaecol Br Cwlth 74 (1967): 812.*

Buller, A.J., and A.C. Dornhorst. "The physics of some pulmonary signs." *The Lancet* (September 1956): 1793-95.

Bunin, N.J., and M.B. Loundon. "Lung sound terminology in case reports." *Chest* 76 (December 1979): 690-92.

Burgess, W.R., and V. Chernick. *Respiratory Therapy in Newborn Infants and Children.* New York: Thieme-Stratton, Inc., 1982.

Cabot, R.C., and H.F. Dodge. "Frequency characteristics of heart and lung sounds." *J.A.M.A.* 84 (1925): 1793-95.

Campbell, E.J.M. *The Respiratory Muscles and the Mechanics of Breathing.* London: Lloyd-Luke, Ltd., 1958.

Carr, R.D. "Skin." In *Physical Diagnosis: The History and Examination of the Patient,* 5th ed., pp. 63-69. Edited by John A. Prior and Jack S. Silberstein. St. Louis: The C.V. Mosby Company, 1977.

Cherniack, R.M., L. Cherniack, and A. Naimark. *Respiration in Health and Disease,* 2nd ed., Philadelphia: W.B. Saunders Company, 1972.

Crofton, J., and A. Douglas. *Respiratory Diseases,* 2nd. ed., Oxford: Blackwell Scientific Publications, Ltd., 1975.

Crutcher, J.C. "Chest Structure." In *Clinical Methods: The History, Physical and Laboratory Examinations,* Vol. 2, pp. 531-33. Edited by H. Kenneth Walker, W. Dallas Hall, and J. Willis Hurst. Boston: Butterworths, 1976.

Crutcher, J.C. "Chest Motion." In *Clinical Methods: The History, Physical and Laboratory Examinations,* Vol. 2, pp. 534-36. Edited by H. Kenneth Walker, W. Dallas Hall, and J. Willis Hurst. Boston: Butterworths, 1976.

Cugell, D.W. "Sounds of the lungs." *Chest* 73 (March 1978): 311-12.

DeGowin, E.L., and R.L. DeGowin. *Bedside Diagnostic Examination,* 3rd ed. New York: Macmillan Publishing Company, 1976.

Dewees, C.B. "Assessment and Classification of the High Risk Neonate." In *High Risk Perinatal Nursing,* pp. 278-293. Edited by Katherine W. Vestal and Carole Ann Miller McKenzie. Philadelphia: W.B. Saunders Company, 1983.

Druger, G. *The Chest: Its Signs and Sounds.* Los Angeles: Humetrics Corporation, 1973.

Dunn, M.I. "The Cardiovascular System." In *Major's Physical Diagnosis,* 8th ed., pp. 358-516. Edited by Mahlon H. Delp and Robert T. Manning. Philadelphia: W.B. Saunders Company, 1975.

Dworetzsky, M. "Immediate Assessment of Acute Respiratory Distress in Asthma." In *The Asthmatic in Trouble,* pp. 11-15. Edited by Thomas L. Petty. Greenwich: CPC Communications, Inc., 1976.

Ertel, P.Y., M. Lawrence, R.K. Brown, and A.M. Stern. "Stethoscope acoustics, I. The doctor and his stethoscope, II. Transmission and filtration patterns." *Circulation* 34 (November 1966): 899-908.

Farzan, S. *A Concise Handbook of Respiratory Diseases.* Reston: Reston Publishing Company, 1978.

Ferris, B.G. "Epidemiology standardization project." *American Review of Respiratory Disease* 118 (December 1978): 7-52.

174

Forgacs, P. "Crackles and wheezes." *The Lancet* 2 (July 1967): 203-5.

Forgacs, P. "The functional basis of pulmonary sounds." *Chest* 73 (March 1978): 399-405.

Forgacs, P., A.R. Nathoo, and H.D. Richardson. "Breath sounds." *Thorax* 26 (1971): 288-95.

Francis, P.B. "Dyspnea, Breathlessness and Shortness of Breath." In *Clinical Methods: The History, Physical and Laboratory Examinations,* Vol. 1, pp. 129-31. Edited by H. Kenneth Walker, W. Dallas Hall, and J. Willis Hurst. Boston: Butterworths, 1976.

Francis, P.B. "Cough and Sputum Production." In *Clinical Methods: The History, Physical and Laboratory Examinations,* Vol. 1, pp. 132-34. Edited by H. Kenneth Walker, W. Dallas Hall, and J. Willis Hurst. Boston: Butterworths, 1976.

Francis, P.B. "Hemoptysis." In *Clinical Methods: The History, Physical and Laboratory Examinations,* Vol. 1, pp. 132-34. Edited by H. Kenneth Walker, W. Dallas Hall, and J. Willis Hurst. Boston: Butterworths, 1976.

Francis, P.B. "Smoking History." In *Clinical Methods: The History, Physical and Laboratory Examinations,* Vol. 2, 1976.

Fraser, R.G., and J.A. Pare. *Organ Physiology: Structure and Function of the Lung.* Philadelphia: W.B. Saunders Company, 1977.

Garner, T.K., and G.M. Duffell. "Terms for lung sounds." *Annals of Internal Medicine* 91 (December 1979): 928.

Green, R.A., and R.F. Johnson. "Pleural Inflammation and Pleural Effusion." In *Textbook of Pulmonary Diseases,* 2nd. ed., pp. 959-82. Edited by Gerald L. Baum. Boston: Little, Brown and Company, 1974.

Green, R.A., and R.F. Johnson. "Pneumothorax." In *Textbook of Pulmonary Diseases,* 2nd ed., pp. 983-95. Edited by Gerald L. Baum. Boston: Little, Brown and Company, 1974.

Guarino, J.R. "Auscultatory percussion of the chest." *The Lancet* (June 1980): 1332-34.

Harvey, W.P. "Gallop Sounds, Clicks, Snaps, Whoops, Honks, and Other Sounds." In *The Heart: Arteries and Veins,* 4th. ed., pp. 255-68. Edited by J. Willis Hurst. New York: McGraw-Hill Book Company, 1978.

Hopkins, H.U. *Leopold's Principles and Methods of Physical Diagnosis,* 3rd. ed. Philadelphia: W.B. Saunders Company, 1965.

Hudson, L.D., R.D. Conn, R.S. Matsubara, and A.H. Pribble. "Roles: diagnostic uselessness of qualitative adjectives." *American Review of Respiratory Disease* 113 (Part 2) (1976): 187.

Hudson, R.P. "Perspectives." In *Major's Physical Diagnosis,* 8th. ed., pp. 1-19. Edited by Mahlon H. Delp and Robert T. Manning. Philadelphia: W.B. Saunders Company, 1975.

Jackson, C.L., and J.F. Huber. "Correlated applied anatomy of the bronchial tree and lungs with a system of nomenclature." *Diseases of the Chest* (July-August 1943): 319-26.

Judge, R.D. "Introduction." In *Methods of Clinical Examination: A Physiologic Approach,* 3rd. ed., pp. 1-16. Edited by Richard D. Judge and George D. Zuidema. Boston: Little, Brown and Company, 1974.

Kampmeier, R.H., and T.M. Blake. *Physical Examination in Health and Disease.* Philadelphia: F.A. Davis Company, 1970.

King, R.C. "The fine art of giving a physical: examining the thorax and respiratory system." *RN (for Managers)* 45-8 1982: 54-63.

Klaus, M.H. and A.A. Fanaroff. *Care of the High-Risk Neonate,* 2nd. ed., Philadelphia: W.B. Saunders Company, 1979.

Kleinerman, J., and H.G. Boren. "Morphologic Basis of Chronic Obstructive Pulmonary Disease: Anatomy of the Tracheobronchial Tree and Lung." In *Textbook of Pulmonary Diseases,* 2nd. ed., pp. 551-78. Edited by Gerald L. Baum. Boston: Little, Brown and Company, 1974.

Kleinerman, J. "Pulmonary Diseases Related to Organic Materials and Radiation." In *Textbook of Pulmonary Diseases,* 2nd. ed., pp. 525-38. Edited by Gerald L. Baum. Boston: Little, Brown and Company, 1974.

Kory, R.C., and J.R. Smith. "Medical History and Physical Examination in the Assessment of Pulmonary Disease." In *Textbook of Pulmonary Diseases,* 2nd. ed., pp. 3-26. Edited by Gerald L. Baum. Boston: Little, Brown and Company, 1974.

Leatham, A. *Auscultation of the Heart and Phonocardiography,* 2nd. ed. London: J & A Churchill, Ltd., 1975.

Leatham, A. "The First and Second Heart Sounds." In *The Heart: Arteries and Veins,* 4th. ed., pp. 237-55. Edited by J. Willis Hurst. New York: McGraw-Hill Book Company, 1978.

Leblanc, P., P.T. Macklem, and W.R.D. Ross. "Breath sounds and distribution of pulmonary ventilation." *American Review of Respiratory Disease* 102 (1970): 10-16.

Lebowitz, M.D. "Occupational exposures in relation to symptomatology and lung function in a community population." *Environmental Research* 14 (1977): 59-67.

Lerch, C., and V. Bliss. *Maternity Nursing,* 3rd. ed., St. Louis: C.V. Mosby Co., 1978.

Leverenz, C.J., and A.H. Skelly. "Assessment of thorax and lungs." *Occupational Health Nursing* 31, No. 6 (1983): 9-16.

Lewis, H.P. *The History and Physical Examination.* New York: Appleton-Century-Crofts, 1979.

Loudon, R.G. "Auscultation of the lung." *Clinical Notes in Respiratory Disease* 21-2 (1982): 3-7.

Louria, D.B. "Bacterial Pneumonia." In *Textbook of Pulmonary Diseases,* 2nd. ed., pp. 163-86. Edited by Gerald L. Baum. Boston: Little, Brown and Company, 1974.

Lucas, D.S. "Dyspnea." In *Signs and Symptoms: Applied Pathologic Physiology and Clinical Interpretation,* 5th. ed., pp. 341-57. Edited by Cyril Mitchell MacBryde and Robert Stanley Blacklow. Philadelphia: J.B. Lippincott Company, 1970.

Lucas, D.S. "Cyanosis." In *Signs and Symptoms: Applied Pathologic Physiology and Clinical Interpretation,* 5th. ed., pp. 358-68. Edited by Cyril Mitchell MacBryde and Robert Stanley Blacklow. Philadelphia: J.B. Lippincott Company, 1970.

Lynch, P.J. "Skin." In *Methods of Clinical Examination: A Physiologic Approach,* 3rd. ed., pp. 53-60. Edited by Richard D. Judge and George D. Zuidema. Boston: Little, Brown and Company, 1974.

McKusick, V.A., J.T. Jenkins, and G.N. Webb. "The Accoustic Basis of the Chest Examination: Studies by Means of Sound Spectrography." *American Review of Tuberculosis and Pulmonary Diseases* 72 (1955): 12-34.

Malasanos, L., V. Barkauskas, M. Moss, and K. Stoltenberg-Allen. *Health Assessment.* St. Louis: The C.V. Mosby Company, 1977.

Manning, R.T., and M.H. Delp. "The Clinical Process." In *Major's Physical Diagnosis,* 8th. ed., pp. 20-87. Edited by Mahlon H. Delp and Robert T. Manning. Philadelphia: W.B. Saunders Company, 1975.

Mazzaferri, E.L. "Head, Face and Neck." In *Physical Diagnosis: The History and Examination of the Patient,* 5th. ed., pp. 70-97. Edited by John A. Prior and Jack S. Silberstein. St. Louis: The C.V. Mosby Company, 1977.

Miller, E. "Chemotactic function in the human neonate: humoral and cellular aspects." *Pediatric Research* 5 (1971): 487.

Mitchell, R.S., and J.A. Pierce. "Cough." In *Signs and Symptoms: Applied Pathologic Physiology and Clinical Interpretation,* 5th. ed., pp. 324-36. Edited by Cyril Mitchell MacBryde and Robert Stanley Blacklow. Philadelphia: J.B. Lippincott Company, 1970.

Morris, D.C. "Orthopnea." In *Clinical Methods: The History, Physical and Laboratory Examinations,* Vol. 1, pp. 158-59. Edited by H. Kenneth Walker, W. Dallas Hall, and J. Willis Hurst. Boston: Butterworths, 1976.

Morris, D.C. "Paroxysmal Nocturnal Dyspnea." In *Clinical Methods: The History, Physical and Laboratory Examinations,* Vol. 1, pp. 160-61. Edited By H. Kenneth Walker, W. Dallas Hall and J. Willis Hurst. Boston: Butterworths, 1976.

Moser, K.M., and R.A. Bordow. "Chronic Obstructive Pulmonary Disease: Definition, Epidemology, and Pathology."

In *Manual of Clinical Problems in Pulmonary Medicine,* pp. 208-13. Edited by Richard A. Bordow, Edward W. Stool, and Kenneth M. Moser. Boston: Little, Brown and Company, 1980.

Murphy, R.L. "Auscultation of the lung: past lessons, future possibilities." *Thorax* 36-2 (1981): 99-107.

Murphy, R.L.H., and S.K. Holford. "Lung Sounds." *Basics of RD,* American Lung Association, Vol. 4, No. 8, (March 1980).

Myerson, R.M. "Spontaneous pneumothorax: clinical study of 100 consecutive cases." *New England Journal of Medicine* 238 (April 1948): 461-63.

Nath, A.R., and L.H. Capel. "Inspiratory crackles - early and late." *Thorax* 29 (March 1974): 223-27.

Nath, A.R., and L.H. Capel. "Inspiratory crackles and mechanical events of breathing." *Thorax* 29 (November 1974): 695-98.

Perera, G.A., and R.W. Berliner. "The relation of postural hemodilution of paroxysmal dyspnea." *Journal of Clinical Investigation* 22 (January 1943): 25-28.

Pierce, J.A. "Hemoptysis." In *Signs and Symptoms: Applied Pathologic Physiology and Clinical Interpretation,* 5th. ed., pp. 337-40. Edited by Cyril Mitchell MacBryde and Robert Stanley Blacklow. Philadelphia: J.B. Lippincott Company, 1970.

Prior, J.A., and J.S. Silberstein. "Medical History." In *Physical Diagnosis: The History and Examination of the Patient,* 5th. ed., pp. 5-11. Edited by John A. Prior and Jack S. Silberstein. St. Louis: The C.V. Mosby Company, 1977.

Prior, J.A., and J.S. Silberstein. "Chief Complaint and Present Illness." In *Physical Diagnosis: The History and Examination of the Patient,* 5th. ed., pp. 12-19. Edited by John A. Prior and Jack S. Silberstein. St. Louis: The C.V. Mosby Company, 1977.

Prior, J.A., and J.S. Silberstein. "Past, Family, Social, and Occupational History and Systems Review." In *Physical Diagnosis: The History and Examination of the Patient,* 5th. ed., pp. 20-35. Edited by John A. Prior and Jack S. Silberstein. St. Louis: The C.V. Mosby Company, 1977.

Prior, J.A. "Thorax and Lungs." In *Physical Diagnosis: The History and Examination of the Patient,* 5th. ed., pp. 187-224. Edited by John A. Prior and Jack S. Silberstein. St. Louis: The C.V. Mosby Company, 1977.

"Pulmonary terms and symbols: A report of the ACCP-ATS joint committee on pulmonary nomenclature." *Chest* 67 (May 1975): 583-93.

Pursel, S.E., and G.E. Lindskog. "Hemoptysis: A clinical evaluation of 105 patients examined consecutively on a thoracic surgical service." *American Review of Respiratory Disease* 84 (September 1961): 329-36.

Rabin, C.B. "New or neglected physical signs in diagnosis of chest diseases." *J.A.M.A.* 194 (November 1965): 158-62.

Rappaport, M.B., and H.B. Sprague. "Physiologic and physical laws that govern auscultation, and their clinical application." *The American Heart Journal* 21 (March 1941): 257-316.

Rarey, K.P., and J.W. Youtsey. *Respiratory Patient Care.* Englewood Cliffs: Prentice-Hall, Inc., 1981.

Ravitch, M.M. "Disorders of the Chest Wall." In *Davis-Christopher Textbook of Surgery, The Biological Basis of Modern Surgical Practice,* 10th ed., pp 1862-71. Edited by David C. Sabiston. Philadelphia: W.B. Saunders Company, 1972.

Robertson, A.J., and R. Coope. "Rales, ronchi, and Laennec." *The Lancet* 2 (August 1957): 417-22.

Robinson, D.W. "Examination of the Head and Neck." In *Major's Physical Diagnosis,* 8th. ed., pp. 175-229. Edited by Mahlon H. Delp and Robert T. Manning. Philadelphia: W.B. Saunders Company, 1975.

Ruth, W.E. "Examination of the Chest, Lungs, and Pulmonary System." In *Major's Physical Diagnosis,* 8th. ed., pp. 301-57. Edited by Mahlon H. Delp and Robert T. Manning. Philadelphia: W.B. Saunders Company, 1975.

Seeds, A., and R. Behrman. "Acid-base monitoring of the fetus during labor with blood obtained from the scalp." *J. Pediatrics* 74 (1969): 804.

Silberstein, J.S. "General Inspection." In *Physical Diagnosis: The History and Examination of the Patient*, 5th. ed., pp. 54-62. Edited by John A. Prior and Jack S. Silberstein. St. Louis: The C.V. Mosby Company, 1977.

Silberstein, J.S. "Cardiovascular System." In *Physical Diagnosis: The History and Examination of the Patient*, 5th ed., pp. 239-97. Edited by John A. Prior and Jack S. Silberstein. St. Louis: The C.V. Mosby Company, 1977.

Silverman, B.D. "Palpitation." In *Clinical Methods: The History, Physical, and Laboratory Examinations*. Vol. 1, pp. 168-69. Edited by H. Kenneth Walker, W. Dallas Hall and J. Willis Hurst. Boston: Butterworths, 1976.

Smyllie, H.C., L.M. Blendis, and P. Armitage. "Observer disagreement in physical signs of the respiratory system." *The Lancet* 289 (August 1965): 412-13.

Stegman, D., and B. Mead. "The chest wall twinge syndrome." *Nebraska Medical Journal* (September 1970): 528-33.

Terr, A.I. "Bronchial Asthma." In *Textbook of Pulmonary Diseases*, 2nd. ed., pp. 421-44. Edited by Gerald L. Baum. Boston: Little, Brown and Company, 1974.

Tuttle, E.P. "Hypertension." In *Clinical Methods: The History, Physical, and Laboratory Examinations*, Vol. 1, pp. 183-85. Edited by H. Kenneth Walker, W. Dallas Hall, and J. Willis Hurst. Boston: Butterworths, 1976.

Walker, H.K., and J.W. Hurst. "The Problem-Oriented Medical Information System." In *Methods of Clinical Examination: A Physiologic Approach*, 3rd. ed., pp. 17-30. Edited by Richard D. Judge and George D. Zuidema. Boston: Little, Brown and Company, 1974.

Ward, J.A. "Neck Inspection." In *Clinical Methods: The History, Physical, and Laboratory Examinations*, Vol. 2, pp. 515-17. Edited by H. Kenneth Walker, W. Dallas Hall, and J. Willis Hurst. Boston: Butterworths, 1976.

Ward, J.A. "Thyroid Examination." In *Clinical Methods: The History, Physical and Laboratory Examination*, Vol. 2, pp. 521-24. Edited by H. Kenneth Walker, W. Dallas Hall, and J. Willis Hurst. Boston: Butterworths, 1976.

Weg, J.G., and R.A. Green. "Respiratory System." In *Methods of Clinical Examination: A Physiologic Approach,* 3rd. ed., pp. 105-40. Edited by Richard D. Judge and George B. Zuidema. Boston: Little, Brown and Company, 1974.

Williams, T.J., D. Ahmed, and W.K. Morgan. "A clinical and roentgenographic correlation of diaphragmatic movement." *Archives of Internal Medicine* 141 (June 1981): 878-80.

# Index

# INDEX

Accidents, 23
Anginal pain, 45
Aspiration
of foreign bodies, 37
Asthma
auscultation, 149
chest radiology, 149-50
definition, 147
history, 147-48
inspection, 148-49
palpation, 149
percussion, 149
Atelectasis
auscultation, 163
chest radiology, 164
compression, 161
definition, 161-62
history, 162
inspection, 162
obstructive, 161
palpation, 162-63
percussion, 163
Atrial gallop, 143
Attitude
(see Professional clinician
attitude)
Auscultation
abnormal breath sounds,
136-38
adventitious sounds, 138-39
asthma, 149
atelectasis, 163
auscultory tones, 129
chronic bronchitis, 155
crackles, 138-39
definition, 129
emphysema, 152
errors in, 133-34
heart sounds, 141-44
immediate, 129
mediate, 129
normal breath sounds,
134-36
pleural effusion, 166-67
pleural friction rub, 139
pneumonia, 158

pneumothorax, 169
pulmonary fibrosis, 161
stethoscope, 130-32
techniques, 132-33
voice sounds, 139-140
wheezes, 139
Auscultory gap, 65-66
Auscultory method, 65

Barrel chest, 90
Biot's breathing, 100
Blood pressure
auscultory gap, 65-66
auscultory method, 65
diastolic pressure, 65
mean arterial pressure, 67
normal findings, 66
overview, 64-65
palpatory systolic pressure,
65
procedure for measuring,
65
pulse pressure, 66-67
sources of error in
measuring, 68
systolic pressure, 65
variations in, 67
Bradycardia, 63
Bradypnea, 99
Breathing
abnormal breath sounds,
136-38
adventitious sounds, 138-39
crackles, 138-39
normal breath sounds,
134-36
pleural friction rub, 139
rate, type, and pattern,
98-100
wheezes, 139
Bronchiectasis, 37
Bronchitis
(see Chronic bronchitis)
Bronchophony, 140

Carcinoma, 37

Cardiopulmonary disease, 39
Cardiopulmonary symptoms
  chest pain, 42-49
  cough, 31-33
  dyspnea, 38-42
  hemoptysis, 35-38
  overview, 31
  sputum, 33-35
  wheezing, 49-51
Cardiovascular disease, 37-38
  sources, 38
Chest
  inspection, 89-90
Chest pain
  character, 47
  characterizing, 46-49
  definition, 42-49
  location, 46
  musculoskeletal pain, 46
  palpitation, 48-49
  pleuritic pain, 43-44
  precordial pain, 42-43
  relieving and aggravating
    factors, 48
  setting, 47-48
  severity, 46-47
  substernal pain, 44-46
  tracheobronchial pain, 43
Chest radiology
  asthma, 149-50
  atelectasis, 164
  chronic bronchitis, 155
  emphysema, 153
  pleural effusion, 167
  pneumonia, 158
  pneumothorax, 169
  pulmonary fibrosis, 161
Cheyne-Stokes respiration,
  99-100
Chief complaint, 17
Childhood diseases, 22
Chronic bronchitis
  auscultation, 155
  chest radiology, 155
  definition, 153-54
  history, 154
  inspection, 154
  palpation, 155
  percussion, 155
Chronic obstructive
  pulmonary disease, 39, 42
Chylothorax, 165
Clinician attitude

(*see* Professional clinician
  attitude)
Continuous fever, 59
Cough
  definition, 31
  mechanism, 31-32
  pulmonary disease, 32
Crackles, 138-39
Crepitations, 112-13
Cyanosis, 75-76

Diaphragmatic excursion,
  124, 126
Diastolic pressure, 65
Digital clubbing, 79-80
Direct question, 7
Dyspnea
  cardiopulmonary disease,
    39
  characterizing, 40-42
  chronic obstructive
    pulmonary disease, 42
  definition, 38, 99
  inspiratory and expiratory,
    39-40
Dysrhythmia, 63

Ectomorphs, 73
Edema, 81
Egophony, 140
Emphysema
  auscultation, 152
  chest radiology, 153
  definition, 150
  history, 150-51
  inspection, 151-52
  palpation, 152
  percussion, 152
  subcutaneous, 112-13
Empyema, 165
Endomorph, 73-74
Examination
  (*see* Physical examination)
Extremities
  digital clubbing, 79-80
  edema, 81
  inspection, 78-81
  nails, 79

Family history, 23-24

Fever
  continuous, 59
  intermittent, 60
  relapsing, 60
  remittant, 60
Fibrosis
  (*see* Pulmonary fibrosis)
Fremitus, 111-12

Galileo, 57

Heart sounds
  atrial gallop, 143
  first, 141
  second, 141-42
  valve areas, 143-44
  ventricular gallop, 142-43
Hemoptysis
  aspiraton of foreign bodies, 37
  bronchiectasis, 37
  carcinoma, 37
  cardiovascular disease, 37-38
  definition, 35-36
  inflammation, 36-37
  trauma, 36
Hemothorax, 165
History of present illness
  course of complaint, 19
  date of onset, 18
  exacerbations, 20
  location of complaint, 19
  nature of complaint, 18-19
  overview, 17-18
  treatment, 20
Hydrothorax, 165
Hyperpnea, 99
Hypopnea, 99

Illnesses, 23
Inflammation, 36-37
Inspection
  asthma, 148-49
  atelectasis, 162
  breathing, 98-100
  chest, 89-90
  chronic bronchitis, 154
  definition, 71

  emphysema, 151-52
  extremities, 78-81
  mental status, 72-73
  neck, 76-78
  nutritional status, 73-74
  performing, 71-72
  pleural effusion, 165-66
  pneumonia, 157
  pneumothorax, 168
  posture, 74
  pulmonary fibrosis, 160
  skin, 74-76
  thorax, 81-85, 88-94, 96-100
Intermittent fever, 60
Interview
  (*see* Patient interview)

Kussmaul breathing, 99
Kyphosis, 93-94

Laennec, 130
Life history, 24-25
Listening, 9-10
Lordosis, 94
Lungs
  crepitations, 112-13
  palpitation, 108, 111-13
  segmental anatomy, 88-89
  thoracic expansion, 108
  vocal fremitus, 111-12

Massive pulmonary
  embolism, 46
Mean arterial pressure, 67
Mesomorphs, 73
Mucus, 33
Muscles of inspiration
  retractions, 96
  use of accessory, 96-97
Musculoskeletal pain, 46

Nails, 79
Neck
  accessory muscles, 78
  inspection, 76-78
  laryngeal cartilages, 78, 103-104
  mobility, 77

palpitation, 103-106
pulsations, 78
scars, 77
size and shape, 76
symmetry, 77
thyroid gland, 104-105
trachea, 106-107
Nonverbal communication, 9
Normal sinus rhythm, 63

Open-ended question, 7
Orthopnea, 40-41

Palpation
asthma, 149
atelectasis, 162-63
chronic bronchitis, 155
crepitations, 112-13
definition, 103
neck, 103-106
pleural effusion, 166
pneumonia, 157
point of maximal impulse, 113
pulmonary fibrosis, 160
skin, 103
thoracic expansion, 108
thorax and lungs, 108, 111-13
thyroid gland, 104-105
trachea, 106-107
vocal fremitus, 111-12
Palpatory systolic pressure, 65
Palpitation, 48-49
Paroxysmal nocturnal dyspnea, 41-42
Past medical history
accidents, 23
childhood diseases, 22
illnesses, 23
overview, 20, 22
previous hospitalizations, 22-23
Patient examination
(*see* Physical examination)
Patient history
chief complaint, 17
education, 25
family history, 23-24

history of present illnesses, 17-18
life history, 24-25
medications, 25-26
occupational history, 25
past medical history, 20, 22-23
personal habits, 26-27
personal history, 24
smoking history, 27-28
socioeconomic status, 25
Patient interview
clinical approach, 3-6
clinician attitude, 4-6
clinician attitude problems, 11-12
communication errors, 12
errors in data collection, 10
initiating the interview, 4
listening, 9-10
overview, 3
pitfalls, 10-12
privacy, 3-4
questioning techniques, 6-9
structure, 10-11
Patient privacy, 3-4
Pectoriloquy
whispered, 140
Pectus carinatum, 90
Pectus excavatum, 90
Percussion
asthma, 149
atelectasis, 163
characteristics of notes, 120-21
chronic bronchitis, 155
definition, 117
diaphragmatic excursion, 124, 126
dull note, 123
duration, 120
emphysema, 152
flat note, 123-24
hyperresonant note, 122
immediate, 118
intensity, 120
location of notes, 121-24
mediate, 118
pitch, 120
pleural effusion, 166
pneumonia, 157-58
pneumothorax, 169

pulmonary fibrosis, 160
quality, 120-21
resonant note, 121-22
techniques, 118-19
tympanic note, 122-23
Personal history, 24
Physical examination
blood pressure, 64-68
examination procedure,
55-56
examination room
environment, 56-57
measuring vital signs, 57
overview, 55
pulse, 62-64
temperature, 57-58
Pleural effusion
auscultation, 166-67
chest radiology, 167
definition, 164-65
history, 165
inspection, 165-66
palpation, 166
percussion, 166
Pleuritic pain, 43-44
Pneumonia
auscultation, 158
chest radiology, 158
definition, 156
history, 156-57
inspection, 157
palpation, 157
percussion, 157-58
Pneumothorax
auscultation, 169
chest radiology, 169
closed, 167-68
definition, 167-68
history, 168
inspection, 168
open, 167
percussion, 169
tension, 168
Point of maximal impulse,
113
Posture, 74
Precordial pain, 42-43
Present illness
(see History of present
illness)
Previous hospitalizations,
22-23

Professional clinician
attitude, 4-6
Pulmonary fibrosis
auscultation, 161
chest radiology, 161
definition, 158-59
history, 159-60
inspection, 160
palpation, 160
percussion, 160
Pulse
abnormalities, 63-64
character, 63
overview, 62
rate, 62-63
rhythm, 63
Pulse pressure, 66-67
Pulsus alternans, 64
Pulsus paradoxus, 64
Pulsus parvus, 63
Pyothorax, 165

Questioning techniques
clinician tone of voice, 6-7
direct question, 7
nonverbal communication,
9
open-ended question, 7
opening the interview, 6
types of questions, 8
use of outline, 6

Relapsing fever, 60
Remittant fever, 60

Scalene muscles, 96-97
Scoliosis, 94
Sighing, 100
Skin
color, 75
cyanosis, 75-76
inspection, 74-76
palpitation, 103
turgor, 103
Smoking history, 27-28
Sputum
characteristics, 35
definition, 33
production, 34-35

Sternocleidomastoid muscles, 97
Stethoscope
  bell, 131
  chest piece, 131-32
  diaphragm chest piece, 132
  earpieces, 130
  tubing, 131
Stridor, 40
Subcutaneous emphysema, 112-13
Substernal pain, 44-46
Symptoms
  definition, 31
Systolic pressure, 65

Tachycardia, 63
Tachypnea, 99
Temperature
  body, 57
  continuous fever, 59
  intermittent fever, 60
  methods for assessing, 58
  normal, 59
  relapsing fever, 60
  remittant fever, 60
Thoracentesis, 165
Thorax
  accessory muscles of inspiration, 96-97
  bony landmarks, 83-84
  chest inspection, 89-90

crepitations, 112-13
deformities, 90, 93-94
lobar anatomy, 84-85
palpitation, 108, 111-13
reference lines, 81-83
segmental anatomy of lungs, 88-89
thoracic expansion, 108
vocal fremitus, 111-12
Thyroid gland
  palpitation, 104-105
Trachea
  palpitation, 106-107
Tracheobronchial pain, 43
Transudate, 164
Trapezius muscles, 97
Trauma, 36

Ventricular gallop, 142-43
Vital signs, 57
Voice sounds, 139-40

Wheezing, 139
  definition, 49-50
  evaluating, 50-51
  expiratory, 50